SLIMNASTICS

THE WHOLE PERSON APPROACH TO FITNESS

Diana Lamplugh & Pamela Nottidge

The Oxford Illustrated Press

Front Cover
Our thanks for the photographs on the cover go to:
Top:
Tony Stone Associates.
Middle:
Les Brazier, Mark Wilkins, Haynes Publishing.
Bottom:
Here's Health magazine.

Exercise Photography
For her patience, hard work and good humour through two long photographic sessions, our thanks must go to Betty Nelson for the modelling of the exercises and Les Brazier and Mark Wilkins for the photography.

© Diana Lamplugh, Pamela Nottidge, 1984
Reprinted, 1984
Printed in Great Britain by
J. H. Haynes & Co Limited
ISBN 0 902280 93 7
The Oxford Illustrated Press, Sparkford,
Yeovil, Somerset BA22 7JJ

Acknowledgements

We are very grateful to all those who have acted as consultants, advisers, and contributors, and would like to thank them for the time, energy, expertise, thought, and encouragement they have given in the preparation of this book.

In particular we would like to thank:

Dr. Peter Mitchell-Heggs, M.A., Ph.D., M.R.C.P.—Harley Street and Epsom

Dr. Nita Mitchell-Heggs, M.B., S.C., M.R.C.P.

Dr. Florence Cadogan, M.B., Bs.Dph., M.F.C.M.—Queen Mary's Hospital

Daphne M. Horder, M.H.C.I.M.A., S.R.D., Cert Health Ed., Community Dietitian, St. George's Hospital, Tooting

for their help on vetting the whole book.

For their specialist expertise and inspiration we would like to thank:

Section 1 Exercise:

Miss P. E. Kennedy, lecturer, writer on anatomy and movement

Billie Leighton and Diana Sterwin, members of the Slimnastics Training Committee and contributors to the Training Manuals for Tutors and Leaders.

Violet Palmer, physiotherapist and physiotherapy teacher, former Vice-President, St. Mary's Hospital of Physical Medicine.

Section 2 Healthy Eating:

Miss Jennifer Keogh, SRD., St. James' Hospital, Balham

Anne Battle, Dip.Ed., Home Ec., and the pupils of the Pembroke School, Flackwell Heath, Bucks.

Jane Knight and the pupils of Moreton Hall School, Oswestry, Salop.

Sian Thomas, SRD., and Slimnastics Leader.

Recipes: Valerie and Sally 'Home Cooking for All Occasions', Ealing

Members of Diana Lamplugh's classes in Ealing and Richmond

Section 3 Relaxation:

J. Macdonald Wallace, Principal Lecturer in Health Education

Penny Yendell, Dip.Phys.Ed., Cert. Ed., Consultant to the Health Education Council

Lady Ruth Lloyd, Slimnastics Leader, Tutor L.A.Y.

Section 4 Life Style:

Dr. Michael Smith, broadcaster and writer, Hon. Chief Medical Officer to the F.P.A.

Margaret Melville L.D.S.

The Health Education Council

A.S.H.

ACCEPT (Alcoholism Community Centres for Education, Prevention and Treatment)

Appendices:

Safeways Food Stores Ltd.

J. Sainsbury P.L.C.

British Nutrition Foundation

We would also like to thank our Slimnastics leaders and the members of their classes who contributed so much enthusiasm and so many ideas as well as carrying through this Slimnastics 'whole person' approach to fitness with such effect. In particular we would like to show our appreciation to the members of Diana's Slimnastics classes under the Ealing Further Education Authority and Richmond Adult College and to Pamela's Slimnastics Leaders Courses at The YMCA, Tottenham Court Road, London, for testing all the ideas in this book with such patience and good humour.

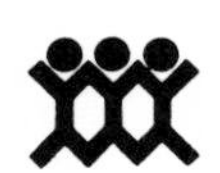

For further information about **The Slimnastics® Organisation,** contact Diana Lamplugh, 14 East Sheen Avenue, London SW14 8AS.
Pamela Nottidge and Diana Lamplugh are both founders of The Slimnastics Organisation.

CONTENTS

Foreword

The Slimnastics Programme
The 'Whole Person' Approach to Fitness

Slimnastics combines Exercise, Healthy Eating, Tension Control, and Living Well. We believe that each aspect of getting fit is interwoven and reliant on the others and that you cannot become truly fit unless you:

- Exercise to keep supple, give stamina, improve your strength and shape as well as help your co-ordination.
- Eat healthily by choosing foods which give energy, keep your body nourished and working well without any extra weight; also cook and serve your meals so they can be eaten with satisfaction and pleasure.
- Practise Tension Control to help avert the physical and mental effects of stress, which together with relaxation aids you to fully appreciate your feelings of well-being as well as cope with any problems and events beyond your control.
- Live a Life Style that allows time for yourself and other people (including holidays and other forms of recreation), not relying on medication, too much alcohol or smoking to alleviate any tension; encouraging consideration of yourself through which you can gain more enjoyment and vitality to enjoy living well.

Slimnastics is being constantly tried, tested and approved by more and more enthusiasts. Apart from the theories, we *know* Slimnastics and its 'whole person' approach to fitness really works in practice . . . we have seen (and our Slimnasts have felt) the results over and over again.

The psychologist Maslow stated, as a result of research over many years into our basic human needs, that it is our physical well-being which is the base stone of our existence and potentiality. He maintained that this sense of well-being together with our other primary needs of air to breathe, a comfortable temperature and water to drink, is essential before we are able to feel more self-confident and able to cope with ourselves and our work, as well as have the energy to want to learn more and look outwards beyond our present position in life and give more thought to others. Taking care of ourselves is an important part of living.

When we hunted our food, ate what we caught or found, thought only of the moment and were exhausted each evening, the human race even though hampered by disease was probably as fit as it could be. We still have accidents and teeth problems, but our health is much improved through knowledge and research. Today, however, the fitness of most of us is far below an 'acceptable' or even 'comfortable' level. We need to take some positive steps towards getting fitter. It is worth it! Not only does getting fit aid the quality and probable quantity of our living days, it also gives a joy and zest to life it is hard to describe though easy to notice both in ourselves and others.

This book is to help you on your way; I have kept it simple, easy to follow and I hope fun to do. You will need to give the programme some thought and time but you will not regret it. I wish you the very best of health!

Diana Lamplugh

INTRODUCTION

The Slimnastics Health Assistance Scheme

You will begin to understand once you read and study the sections on Exercise, Eating and Relaxation how much influence you can have over yourself in attaining a good level of fitness and how much this benefits your general state of health and prospects for the future. In fact, barring accident, catastrophe or unseen calamity you can choose to be as fit as you are able and as fit as you need to be for the role you play in life.

Fitness has been described as 'the ability to carry out daily tasks efficiently with enough energy left over to enjoy leisure time pursuits and meet unforeseen emergencies'. A certain level of fitness is necessary for everyone to prevent the deterioration of their organic functions and to keep their bodies working properly and efficiently. Beyond that it depends on your own personal requirements of daily life or your personal preference. For most of us our way of life does not automatically ensure us a good standard of physical fitness, many of us have to change considerably the way we eat, live, work and play. It is in your own hands to give yourself a Personal Assistance Scheme towards Good Health . . . the choice is yours!

INTRODUCTION

What is Fitness?

Recognising your Fitness Level
The level of fitness you are potentially able to achieve is affected by your basic general health, body type, age, sex and inherited factors, whilst your actual fitness is the degree to which that realisable fitness has been fulfilled or developed or harmed by your life style and activities. The components of fitness are:

Body composition The fat content of the body, its shape, proportions and weight-to-size ratio.

Flexibility The range of movements at each joint. This is determined by the mobility of the joints, tendons and ligaments and muscle power which controls them.

Cardiovascular and Respiratory (CVR Fitness) The primary factor in overall fitness that describes how well the heart and lungs supply the active muscles with oxygen and remove waste products.

Muscular Endurance The length of time particular groups of muscles can continue to perform a certain task.

Muscular Strength The maximum force a muscle, or muscle group can apply in one contraction. This is closely related to muscular power, and in general is slow and precise.

Other Factors Fitness is also affected by motor abilities such as co-ordination, balance, agility, reaction time, speed of movement and power as well as the quality of material available for use as energy. It is also affected by the efficiency of the liver and kidney in maintaining an efficient and correct supply and removal of metabolic 'building blocks' and waste products— they cannot do this if they are sullied by toxic material intake.

Usual Causes of Being Unfit

Inactivity is a primary cause – without activity the body tissues waste and physical capacity declines . . . you need exercise.

Eating too little of the right foods so that you lack the vitamins and minerals to keep you alive and lively and the dietary fibre to expel the toxins . . . you need unrefined cereals, fruit, vegetables, nuts and low-fat proteins.

Overeating a) foods which add little but energy value to your diet. These can not only cut down your intake of the right foods but also lead to excessive consumption of energy for the rate of activity and this extra energy is stored as fat . . . you need to cut down on fatty foods and sugary foods.

b) eating too many calories for your own particular metabolic rate. If you are overweight although eating a healthy diet it is essential to cut down on the high calorie foods such as those containing natural sugars (fruit, especially dried fruit) and vegetable oils (nuts) or fish oil (herrings, mackerel, etc.). If you are overweight for your height you are unfit – eating too many calories leads to an accumulation of potential energy which when unused also turns to fat.

Tension caused by overstress wastes the body's physical and mental resources, draining the energy necessary for efficient activity . . . you need tension control and relaxation.

Straining the System or being over-active for the realisable fitness (such as sudden or prolonged exercise), leads to a general 'running down' of the abilities of mind and body. The same effect is shown by the 'exhaustion' experienced by those who are continually under tension.

Life Style by such destructive habits as tobacco smoking (in any form), drinking too much alcohol, a dissipated life style, poorly balanced diet, lack of sleep and insufficient medical care . . . you need to exercise some self control.

Recognising Signs of Unfitness
If you are unfit you may experience:

A general feeling of being run down; that everything is too much trouble; you may constantly avoid physical (and mental) effort.

Breathlessness and a pounding heart after a short burst of exercise such as running for a bus.

Backache because of insufficient support from weak muscles of the back and abdomen.

Bad posture through laziness, fatigue, lack of physical awareness or psychological depression.

Sleep problems because mental activity is unbalanced by physical activity or simply because insufficient energy is used to feel tired; conversely because of overtiredness and inability to cope.

Aching muscles after activities such as walking upstairs or carrying shopping.

Excess weight and too high a percentage of body fat.

The Slimnastics Health Assistance Scheme involves the whole of you and should include:

- A few minutes Slimnastics exercises, daily, and another form of exercise once/twice a week.
- Eating regular meals and following the Slimnastics Healthy Eating Programme on page 56.
- Practising the skill of Tension Control.
- Giving yourself some consideration – living well.

We aim to help you *feel* good! Feeling better is a step forward and helps you on your way to getting fit.

Exercise is Good for You!

There is as yet no machine which can achieve so many versatile movements as the human body; the actions are intricate, dynamic, precise, strong, graceful, accurate, delicate, powerful – the list is infinite and yet we often neglect to make proper use of our bodies and sometimes hardly move at all. We may feel quite content and well enough leading our sedentary, physically idle lives but we must not mislead ourselves – out bodies were made to move, we need to move in order to function properly, indeed we *must* move if we are to realise our full potential and quality of life.

However, just to move without thought or purpose will not normally achieve the best results. When we were children we could usually romp around naturally, keeping our bodies supple, utilising our energy, getting warm and out of breath, testing our strength and ability and stretch, practising our skill and agility, releasing our tension through complete relaxation. You have only to watch pupils in a school playground to remember this; you will see ball games, tag, skipping competitions, jumping, leaping, running and playing – and the occasional child who is just totally oblivious to everyone and in a world of his own.

As adults we often lose this ability to forget the thoughts and problems of our daily lives through the sheer joy of moving and living. Our bodies reflect our moods, feelings, and thoughts – watch people shopping and you will see the tight jawline, the anxious frown, the depressed droop and the sagging shoulders. Our bodies will reveal neglect and misuse; the hooked shoulder from carrying a bag, the unbalanced posture assumed to cope with an injury which has long since healed, stiff joints and slack abdomens. The internal muscles also suffer from lack of use, or hard treatment through poor diet, constipation, being overweight, or perhaps because of a difficult childbirth.

Adults need to take special care when taking the exercise we so badly need. If we take exercise properly we can do ourselves nothing but good; but thoughtlessly approached our expended energies can land us in needless and uncomfortable trouble. Badly tutored so-called 'aerobic' classes swell the queues of patients for the osteopaths and this is hardly surprising as many of these classes start at the wrong end of the exercise pattern.

To ensure complete safety as well as maximum efficiency, exercises should use muscles and joints in the ways for which they were designed and should start from a perfectly balanced position. If you are already supple and mobile and have sufficient leisure time to take a four to five mile jog each morning (or half an hour continuous steady swim) and then do a stretching workout at a slow strong speed, followed by a gentle slowing down into full relaxation, you do not need a Slimnastics Exercise Programme as you will be already achieving the results. This Slimnastics Exercise Programme is for the average person who needs exercise but is lax about taking it and this probably means most of us!

However, **exercise alone is not enough**. The fuel you feed your body affects your health, energy level, body weight and perhaps even state of mind. If you fail to give yourself the right foods in the correct quantities and prepared in the best way to preserve the nutrients, you may be either unwell, undernourished or overweight and almost certainly unfit. The Slimnastics Healthy Eating Programme is therefore just as important as exercise.

Nor will you be fit enough to exercise if you are tense and overstressed (although exercise is a form of positive relaxation). If you start with taut muscles you are in danger of tearing them – therefore you also need the Slimnastics Relaxation Programme.

Similarly exhaustion and tiredness sap your vitality, smoking dramatically affects your physical performance and alcohol acts as a depressant and numbs the senses. Other forms of self-abuse affect you physically too – so your Life Style is equally vital to your ability to move and exercise.

Eating is Good For You!

To stay alive we must eat. Human beings, like animals, depend for life on eating food which usually consists of a combination of plants, flesh, and produce from other animals or fish, who themselves have thrived on plant food. Plants, unlike animals, have the ability to use the energy from sunlight, the carbon dioxide in the atmosphere and water and minerals in the soil to build up complex substances. In this way the energy of sunlight is stored as chemical energy which man consumes and then converts into energy to keep him alive and lively.

During life, our energy is continually and rapidly expended in all living processes – such as the maintenance of body temperatures, heart beat, breathing, digestion and in physical and mental activity. Between meals the energy supply is obtained from body tissues and this has to be restored by food. Regular eating is therefore an essential part of our lives; it is also an enjoyable as well as often social activity. However, it has only recently been fully realised how much it matters to our well-being that we eat the right foods – ones which actively contribute towards our good health – and that these must be in correct proportions as well as suitable quantities, for our own metabolism.

The mechanics of the body may have changed little since primitive man but there has been a drastic change in our way of life as well as in our methods of producing food, the range of choice, and our ability to save physical effort in bringing it to the table. In some ways our diet has been a major factor in improving aspects of our health, but on the other hand many of the diseases of our modern society are being attributed to faults in the national diet. Some authorities have gone so far as to suggest that thirty per cent of the annual deaths from cancer are attributable to diet-related diseases.

Dental caries and peridontal disease are the most common diseases affecting Western man. In England and Wales the prevalence of caries in adults is 98% and a National Survey conducted in 1968 found that only 3 people in 1000 had 28 or more teeth present and free from decay. Dental caries and gum disorders are caused when the sugar contained in foods reacts with the bacteria found in plaque which forms on teeth to cause acids. This attacks the enamel of the teeth and can eventually destroy the fibrous connections between the gums and tooth.

The average present-day British diet reflects that of other Western countries; it includes a high proportion of fat and refined sugar, rather too much salt, some dietary fibre from fruits and vegetables (but relatively little from cereals), and an increasing proportion of alcohol. This is in sharp contrast to the diet of non-affluent countries in which there is a much smaller proportion of fat and sugar, a larger amount of fibre from cereal and vegetable, and relatively little salt.

Non-affluent countries have many problems including diseases and these are not only the diseases of poverty but also those which like 'Western' diseases may be genetically determined. However, studies of disease patterns reveal that certain diseases which are rare in the non-affluent countries occur frequently among affluent peoples. Some of these such as coronary heart disease, diabetes, high blood pressure and diseases of the large bowel (appendicitis, cancer and diverticulitis) can be avoided, prevented or appeased by a change in life style and eating habits.

To give ourselves the maximum chance to be fit and healthy we would do well to concentrate on:

- More unrefined cereals.
- More vegetables of all kinds.
- More fruits.
- More poultry, fish and pulses.
- Leaner meats.
- Cutting out cheese, fat on meat and fried foods.
- Less invisible fats in pâté, tinned foods, made up meats, cakes, biscuits, puddings, pastry and ice cream.
- Less added sugar and salt (preferably none added at all).

We need a NEW LOOK to our regular eating pattern, Instead of basing our meals around meat, we should think first of cereals and vegetables with the *addition* of a smaller-than-usual portion of meat, fish or cheese (or substitute this with vegetable protein such as pulses or nuts), and should finish with fresh fruit or perhaps a low-fat yoghurt. This may entail changing menu planning, food buying patterns, methods of cooking and altered proportions as well. Quite a number of new thoughts. We believe that eating well will not leave you feeling deprived or losing out on the best things of life, as do some of the recent dieting regimes. On the contrary, eating will be a new experience, satisfying, delicious and full of adventure and fun.

Once again eating well is not enough to ensure good health. You need to *exercise* in order to properly balance the intake and output of calories. *Tension* may well affect your gastric juices and your digestion; over or under eating as well as bingeing are also common reactions to stress; both smoking and alcohol affect the balance of vitamins in the body. All aspects of health are inter-related and combine together to keep you fit; your *life style* cannot be neglected either.

INTRODUCTION

Tension is Good for You!

Without some tension in your body you would be unable to breathe, think, see, speak, keep upright, be lively or alert. Your muscles need some 'tone' to support your skeleton; you also need the stimulation of the brain and hormones to help you to see, think, talk, react and anticipate. Some stress may be good for you in order to heighten your feelings and enjoyment of life.

It is however when the stress causes constant tension or when the stress is too much to stand and the emotional reaction is intense or prolonged, that tension can be the cause not only of behavioural problems but also result in actual physical harm. At the very least it may interfere with your performance or happiness in life. Learning to control this tension is a life-enhancing skill.

Attempts have been made to relate the likelihood of a heart attack to a personality type. Researchers have divided male subjects into two groups: Type A and Type B. Type A have a chronic sense of time-urgency, are aggressive, ambitious, and may drive themselves on to meet (often self imposed) deadlines. They are self-demanding, often doing two or three things at once, impatient and always in a hurry. They are likely to react with hostility to anything that seems to get in their way and are temperamentally incapable of letting up. They are also likely to think they are indispensable. This adds up to a state of constant stress. Type B men exhibit the opposite characteristics: they are less competitive, less preoccupied with achievement, less rushed and generally more easy-going, not allowing their lives to be governed by deadlines. They are better at separating work from play and know how to relax. They are less prone to anger, and do not feel constantly impatient, rushed and under pressure. The incidence of heart attacks is much higher in Type A than in Type B individuals.

However, most people are a mixture of both A and B and in some persons the real mix of A and B might not be immediately apparent. Also as you will see from the physiological responses to stress it is quite possible for a chemical reaction to occur even though there has been no visible bodily sign that any tension has taken place. The human body is a very complex and, in many areas still undiscovered or not understood, territory. You may not feel in need of tension control, you may feel completely relaxed, or you may think that you have not got the time to waste. However, do not let yourself be fooled; everyone can benefit from learning the Tension Control Technique (TCT) and it will stand you in good stead all your life.

Once again it must be remembered that relaxation and tension control on their own are not enough – exercise is almost essential for draining away excess emotion or stress reaction; physical fitness affects your mental ability to cope with tension and stress; eating well is very important. Smoking is a stimulant, drugs and alcohol affect the concentration and the other functions of the brain; the right Life Style for you is also your aim.

Living Well is Good for You!

Our life style does matter to our general health. It is easy to think that if we exercise correctly and frequently, are careful to eat a healthy diet and do not seem to suffer from tension, that we will be able to get away with being overweight, drinking, general self neglect and even smoking without suffering any ill effects. This may well seem overstated when we are young because it takes many years before these forms of self-abuse take their toll.

Smoking tobacco has an effect on physical fitness from the outset, although it takes ten to fifteen years before the effects are so serious that the smoker is likely to die from cancer, heart disease or bronchitis. Perhaps the fact that smoking affects others is even more telling. We can no longer justify our habit by saying: 'Well, if I want to die that way, it's my business', when we are aware that our children and our partners are almost equally affected. Smoking cigarettes can lethally pollute the atmosphere. There is no way we can equate it with health.

Obesity is unsightly and may also be a killer or a contributory factor in diseases. There are many reasons for being very overweight but sometimes it is just due to the fact that we are eating too much of the wrong foods. Eating healthily may be all that is needed; some people will need to take more drastic measures. It is impossible to be obese and truly fit, but on the other hand losing any excess weight will improve your looks, posture, mobility, endurance, strength, shape, breathing and general outlook on life. It is worth it.

Drinking too much alcohol impairs the brain as much as the body. In the 'ACCEPT' (Alcoholism Community Centres for Education, Prevention and Treatment) brochures it states: 'Alcoholism is now our third major health hazard, after heart disease and cancer'. Continued alcohol misuse may lead to social, legal, domestic, job and financial problems. It may also cut a lifespan by ten to fifteen years and lead to overdosing and suicide, accidents and death from drunken driving. Alcohol should always be drunk in moderation.

It is important we take care of ourselves and make sure we do not needlessly run risks through drug or medicine misuse, accidents, lack of hygiene or lack of knowledge. It is also imperative that we make time to give ourselves some consideration. This is not just self-interest. All of us can have some effect on someone. If we are fit, well and relaxed we can look outwards and care for other people as well.

This is the fourth link in the circle without which it would not be complete. By now you must be considering that this Whole Person approach to fitness makes sure that you have a very busy life! However, once you have absorbed it you will discover that it is in fact a way of life and that the exercises, eating, tension control, relaxation and self expectation will become just part of your daily living. However combined these elements will improve not only your physical but also your mental energy. You can put this to good advantage and make more time to enjoy living. We only live this life once and it is not our intention that your healthy life style should feel dull and boring!

SECTION 1

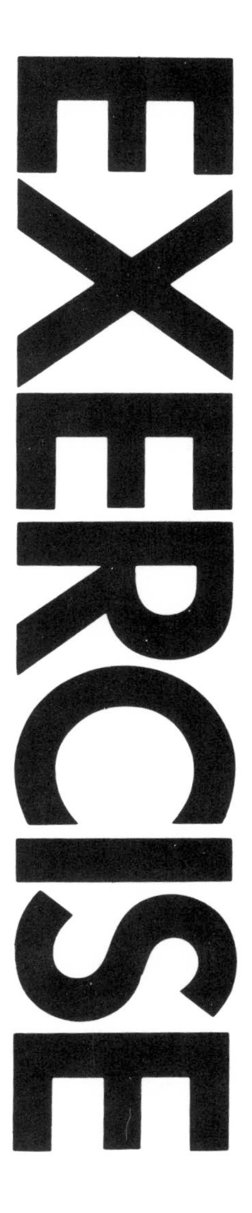

The Slimnastics Exercise Programme

When you do exercises properly, from the correct position and in the right order, your body will respond easily and willingly, with few after effects except that you will look better, feel good and move more easily. These are our aims in Slimnastics.

Slimnastics Exercises follow this pattern:

Posture In Slimnastics we adhere to the saying that 'every movement begins in posture and ends in posture'. Before beginning any exercise, the starting position (i.e. posture) must be as correct as possible, the body balanced and ready to move in the right direction and without danger.

Mobilisation of the Joints These exercises increase the suppleness of the body gradually improving the ability of each joint to move through its full range, and also gently stretch the muscles to prepare the body for more strenuous work. It is essential to stimulate the circulation and lubricate the joints before any other movements. This section is gentle, rhythmical and stretching.

Endurance Section This section includes CVR (Cardio/Vascular/Respiratory) exercises which help improve the heart, circulation and breathing by increasing the pulse rate. These are the exercises which are technically called 'aerobic' (with oxygen). These exercises increase your stamina and help to put up the metabolic rate which is necessary when trying to continue to lose weight on a decreased calorie intake. This section is continuous with a fairly brisk pace.

Strength and Stretch These stronger exercises improve muscle power and tone, giving the quality of firmness, shape and resilience. Before attempting this section the body must be warm and relaxed. The exercises are slow and strong with maximum relationship between movements. Many full-range exercises are used so that the muscles are either fully stretched or fully contracted.

Co-ordination These exercises are designed to improve skill and agility and although they are inter-related with the mobility, endurance and strengthening and stretching exercises, these are specifically to help the neuromuscular co-ordination so important for efficient performance and ability to progress without strain.

The Cool Down This section is important to return the body to its normal state and is achieved by the same exercises as in the mobilisation, using a slow continuous rhythm, and further gentle stretching exercises.

All you need to do is – DO IT! To persuade you, we explain briefly how these exercises work on your body.

EXERCISE

Exercise and the Body

Mobility Exercises for Suppleness (Mobilisation)

Our bones could not work together to transmit body weight and move our body unless they were in some way linked; this occurs through our joints and ligaments. Joints are the places where bone meets bone; some are movable, some immovable. Immovable joints like those of the skull, cushion our bones against breakage caused by blows; movable joints allow bones to move smoothly against each other without damage due to grating. Bones are linked at joints by ligaments; bands of flexible tissue. Torn or overstretched ligaments cause sprains and strains.

Flexibility (or mobility) is the ability of a skeletal joint to move through its full range of movement. The normal range of joint movement is maintained by activities and exercises performed in full range. When the range of movement is limited, rhythmical swinging exercises and gentle pressing movements at the limit of the range help to increase it.

Under normal conditions joint movements are usually limited by tension of the opposing muscles, contact of soft tissues or tension of ligaments. If the constant tightness of the muscle is too much and the body overweight, joint stiffness can occur causing muscular weakness, pain and limited movement. Slimnastics exercises will not only improve joint mobility they will also strengthen weak and flabby muscles and reduce tension.

Mobility exercises should be done at an unhurried relaxed tempo and the increased range of mobility and flexibility should be coaxed not forced. Your breathing should be free and easy to fit the rhythm of the movement.

The benefits which you can experience from these Mobility Exercises are:

- Increased suppleness.
- Gentle strengthening of weak and flabby muscles and a reduction of tension.
- Less aches and pains.
- A more youthful appearance.

Endurance Exercises for Stamina (Pulse-up)

Endurance exercises are a vital part of Slimnastics fitness and are very rewarding physically and mentally. A regular progressive endurance exercise programme is usually accompanied by an increase in:

- The circumference of the muscles as well as 'tone' (slight shortening). The decrease in measurements noted by Slimnasts is due to loss of fat which is very bulky compared to muscle.
- The number of capillaries per unit muscle mass.
- The size and capacity of the heart making it a more efficient pump resulting in a higher maximal pulse rate after exercise, but a slower resting heart rate with a maintained or increased cardiac output – because the more efficient heart pumps more blood per beat.
- The general efficiency of the body and decrease of the recovery period (during which the 'oxygen debt' is paid off), and reduction of fatigue resulting from the exercise.

You should start endurance exercises slowly, and gradually increase the effort and repeats over several weeks.

When you are doing a full exercise programme of endurance exercises progress by decreasing the rest periods between exercises and also by increasing the number of times the exercise is performed. Repetition should not exceed 10/20 times and endurance exercises must be followed by a short period of relaxation.

The benefits you can experience from the Endurance Exercises are:

- Increased energy and stamina.
- Help with continuation of weight loss or maintaining the correct body weight.
- A clearer brain due to oxygen increase.
- A boost to your morale.

Exercises which Strengthen the Muscles (Tone-up)

In static exercise (isometrics) the muscles contract against resistance keeping a joint fixed in one position; for instance by pushing against another person or object, or by opposing two parts of the body. These exercises are good for strengthening muscle around stiff or painful joints but not so good for increasing heart and lung efficiency and so are not enough on their own to promote fitness. It is essential not to hold these exercises for long and to keep breathing regularly thoughout the exercises.

In dynamic exercises the limbs are moved rhythmically. The larger the muscles and more vigorous the effort, the greater the demand for oxygen in the blood and the better the exercise is for the heart and lungs. Therefore for real fitness activities involving dynamic exercise of the legs, they are most effective.

A certain amount of strength is necessary to maintain your posture as well as for your performance of any exercise or daily task so that strength development is an important part of an exercise programme in order to improve results as well as the shape of your body. All voluntary muscles can work from the position in which they are fully stretched to the position in which they are fully contracted and have the dual power of contraction and relaxation. (Living groups of muscle never become completely relaxed, but are constantly in a condition of slight contraction which is known as muscle tone).

The muscles work best when they have become warmed by the endurance of the exercise session. They also stretch most effectively when at rest such as lifting your leg and stretching your ham strings when lying on your back. You should focus your attention on the muscles being stretched, holding a relaxed sustained stretch for between 10-30 seconds before getting on to a point where a mild tension can be felt. These exercises should be done slowly with no bouncing or jerking.

The benefits you can experience by doing these Strengthening Exercises are:

- A better shape.
- Good posture.
- Stronger muscles to support and protect your back.

Co-ordination Exercises for Balance (Fun-up)

Good co-ordination is essential in order to perform not only the Mobility, Endurance and Strengthening Exercises with maximum skill and efficiency but also daily tasks of both body and mind. They are important to ensure good balance and posture and therefore the ability to live without strain.

Co-ordination exercises involve all types of movement and include exercises with equipment and partners as well as emphasis on repetition and sequence. Continual progress can be made, and good results obtained. It is the nervous system which is being exercised!

The benefits you can experience from doing these Balance Exercises are:

- Quicker reactions.
- Faster mental responses.
- Better logical thought.

Posture is Vital

This section is so important, to ensure correct movements, we have gone into the starting positions in more detail.

To maintain the correct posture, whilst performing various exercises and carrying out everyday movements, is one of the important aims of Slimnastics exercises. A balanced skeletal frame ensures that muscles use energy economically. Unbalanced posture wastes energy and sets up stresses that strain tissues and cause pain. Using the body efficiently involves transmitting its weight so that the line of thrust runs centrally through the joints. Before we start exercising it is important to find out what this means in practice.

Lying

Lying supine (on the back) is the easiest of the fundamental positions as the body can be completely supported and is as stable as possible. The muscle work is minimal on a firm, hard surface. In the relaxed body the head naturally rolls to one side, the lumbar spine hollows slightly, the legs roll outwards. (This is less easy on a soft surface such as a spring mattress, which gives way to the contours of the body and supports it.)

Often people find the idea of lying to perform an exercise unfamiliar and difficult. It is, however, an especially good starting position for the very fit. These are the people who are most often constantly standing or moving from the upright position. This involves gravity pulling in one direction only. The gravity pull in lying causes the circulatory, digestive and nervous system to increase the blood supply and thus invigorates and gives a different feel to the body.

If you find lying uncomfortable, this may be due to the lazy stiff joints used to mattresses, armchairs, carpets and so on. The realignment of the body on the hard, straight, firm floor is a beneficial position in itself. It improves body awareness, and accentuates postural faults and tense muscles or stiff joints. However, the benefits will be a new feeling of health, body firmness, confidence and improved posture.

The posture of lying prior to doing an exercise is:

- A stabilised head, eyes looking at the ceiling, neck stretched.
- Shoulders relaxed, arms by the side, hands rolled outwards.
- Abdominal muscles firm to support the spine.
- Knees and inner borders of the feet held together.

A small pillow under the neck or the knees can help to make the position more comfortable for some people.

There are too, many people who may find the lying position difficult or very uncomfortable. It may also be unsuitable if you are obese, elderly or very unfit. In this case you can sit on a chair and adapt the exercises accordingly.

Sitting

This is a comfortable, natural and very stable position. In sitting, the lateral and rotatory movements of the pelvis are eliminated by the weight of the body and position of the legs. So side bending and twisting movements can be localised to the spine. It is therefore excellent for spine mobility. Many hip, knee, and foot and arm exercises can be performed in this position, without the body weight and lack of balance hindering the movements. It is a very good position for correct alignment and posture of the upper part of the body.

Ideally the chair should be firm and upright, with a flat seat, wide enough and long enough to support the thighs fully with the feet resting on the ground. If however, the chair seat is too low, sit with the thighs fully supported and the knees slightly extended. If the seat is too high, sit forward with the feet in firm contact with the floor.

Some Slimnastics Exercises are done in this position with emphasis on correct sitting posture.

The Correct Position for Sitting The pelvis is anchored securely, sitting slightly forward in the middle of the chair seat and your weight evenly divided between the 'sitting bones' (which can be felt if you gently push down onto the chair); stretch tall through the top of your head remembering that your neck is part of your spine and should balance directly above it; rotate the shoulders backwards and then rest the arms and hands on the thighs in a relaxed position; the thigh bones should be parallel or pressed together (depending on the exercise) but the feet should always be flat on the floor and the knees following the same direction as your toes.

Kneeling

Because the centre of gravity is slightly lower, this position is rather more stable than that of standing, and movements of the spine are a little easier to control with more precise movements of the lower trunk and hip joint. This position can teach you the control necessary to achieve a good standing position.

The body should be supported on the knees which may be together or slightly apart. Feet should be 'planter flexed' (pointed). The rest of the body is held as in standing. The lower leg should be relaxed, the body stabilised on the knees by the strong working of the extensors of the hips and flexors of the lumbar spine.

If this position is uncomfortable, knee padding can be made by cutting out the sleeves of an old cardigan which can then be used as leg warmers folded down from the thigh and up from the calf so as to make a triple thickness. A mat or length of foam rubber or cushion can also be used to soften the floor.

Standing

This is the most difficult starting position to maintain as the whole body must be balanced and stabilised in correct alignment on a small base (your feet) by the co-ordinated work of many muscle groups. This is the hardest position in which to achieve pure precise movement and the easiest in which to produce postural faults.

Here is a simple way to check your own individual posture from standing. Feet slightly apart (they will naturally turn out a little), sway forward onto the toes, then backwards onto the heels, now find a comfortable slightly swaying position in the middle, which gives alternate muscle work and rest period to the front and back of the lower leg. Now to the pelvic tilt, which is the key as this alters the position of the spine as a whole. Try the following:

Keep the feet firmly on the ground as described above, now rotate the legs outwards firmly – draw a face on each knee cap then make the faces turn slightly away from each other – this immediately improves the posture of the feet.

Now for altering the posture of the spine, put your hands on the bones of the pelvis on either side of the tummy – tilt the pelvis by sticking your bottom out. Now reverse the tilt which flattens the back and tightens the abdominal muscles. Move the pelvis into mid-tilt so that the correct balance and weight of the body is passing through your knees and just in front of your ankles. Stretch your spine up through your neck to your head, eyes facing forwards, chin at right angles; pull your shoulders down and relax them. Keep breathing gently with your rib cage lifted slightly and your arms relaxed by your sides. To start with, this correct posture might feel tiring and uncomfortable, but the more you practise it the more natural it will feel.

Do this carefully and you will be standing correctly with no undue strain.

20 Guidelines to Exercising Well

Before You Begin Exercising

1. Check with your doctor if you have had any recent, persistent or constant problems with your health or body (i.e. flu, back, hernia, blood pressure, diabetes, heart).

2. Check your environment to make sure it is well ventilated, comfortably heated and not too crowded with obstacles or dangerous in any way (i.e. the floor isn't slippery or full of splinters).

3. Wear the right clothes so that you are able to move freely and not feel constricted in any way.

4. Wear the correct footwear to avoid slipping. Bare feet are excellent if the floor is good. Otherwise cushion your joints and protect yourself from accidents by wearing gym shoes, dance or specially designed non-slip, soft-soled plimsolls.

Before You Start Your Exercises

5. Check your posture. Good posture means better efficiency of the muscles and joints, and internal organs. Remember that added weight affects the posture, puts pressure on the joints, strains the muscles, distorts the internal organs and affects the circulation. So take extra care if this applies to you.

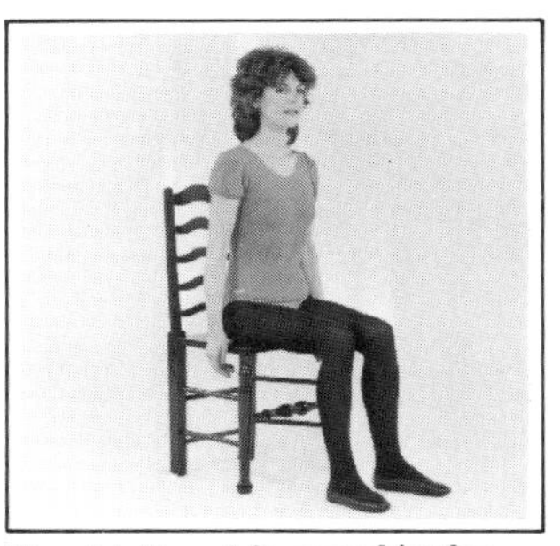

Do sit tall and forward in the chair with feet firmly on the ground.

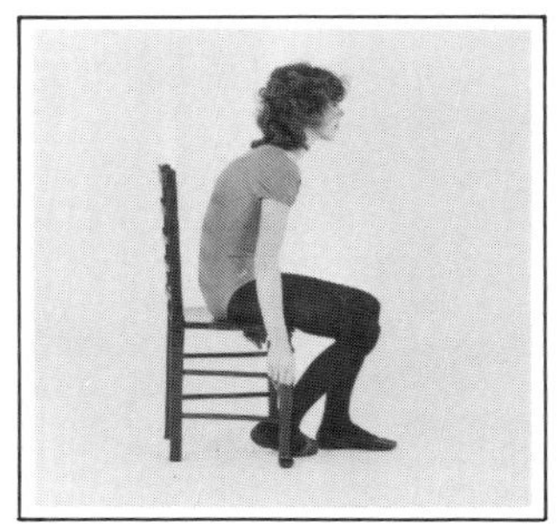

Do not slouch with rounded back, legs crossed.

6. Think tall. Give yourself constant reminders to 'sit up', 'stand up', 'stretch the neck up to the top of the head'. This will not only help ensure that you do the exercises properly but will also prevent tension and exhaustion.

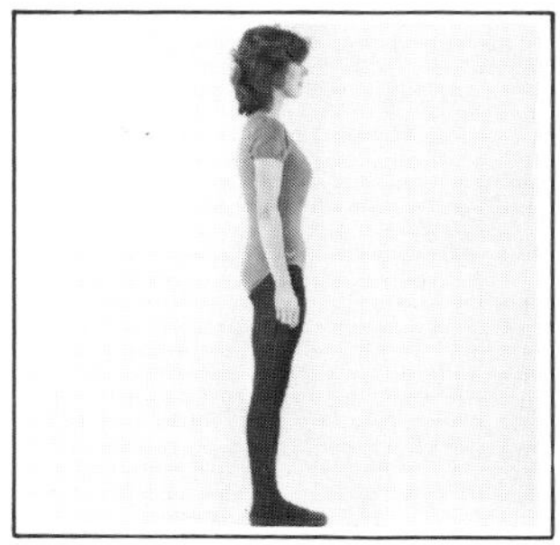

Do stand tall.

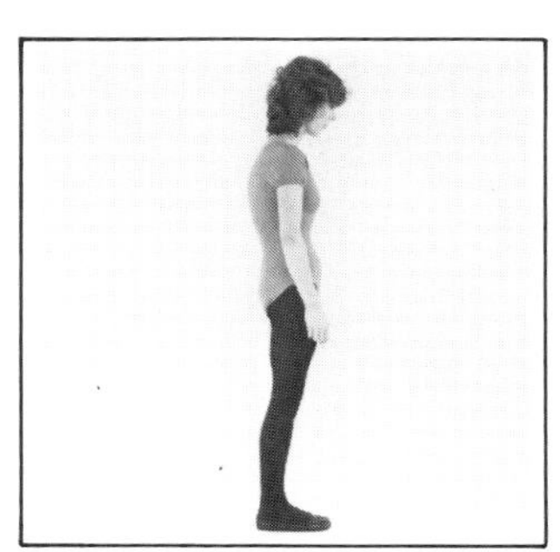

Do not slouch.

7. Remember to keep breathing! Breathe naturally and easily throughout. Holding your breath raises the blood pressure and can cause other problems as well, such as hernias.

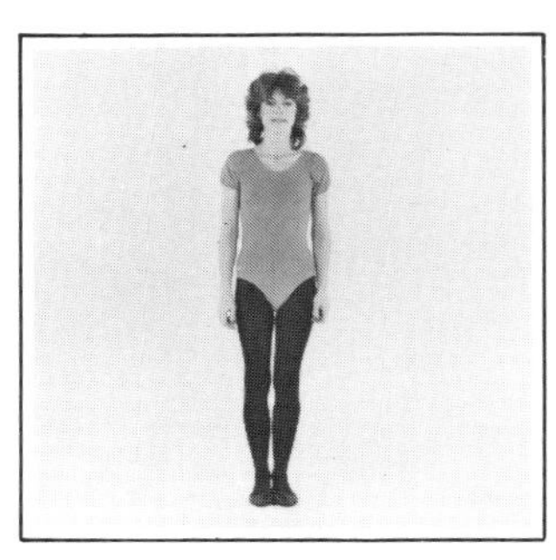

Do keep breathing naturally throughout.

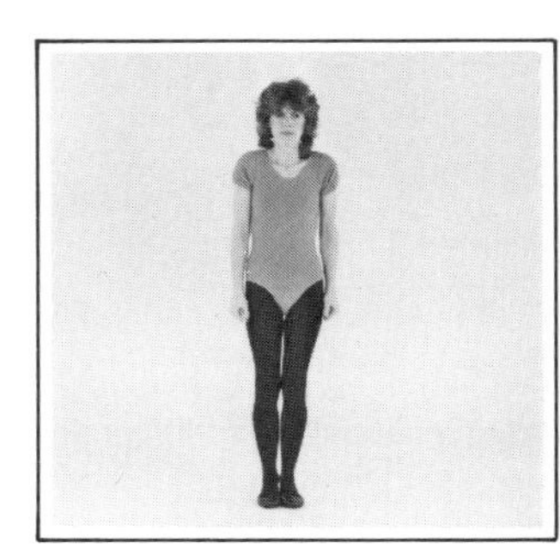

Do not hold your breath.

When You Begin Your Exercises

8. Sit on a chair or lie on the floor to start exercising. However fit you are as an adult warm up the joints and muscles with your body weight supported. This will prevent injury and give your body a better chance for safe fitness. Incorrect movements are often unrecognised when you are standing; sitting or lying are simpler.

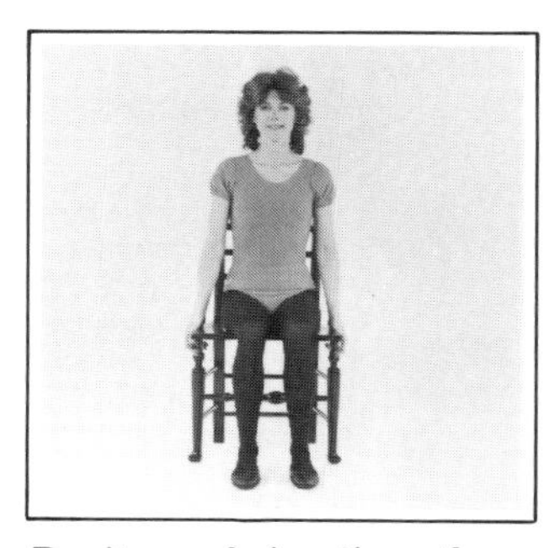

Do sit on a chair or lie on the floor to start exercising.

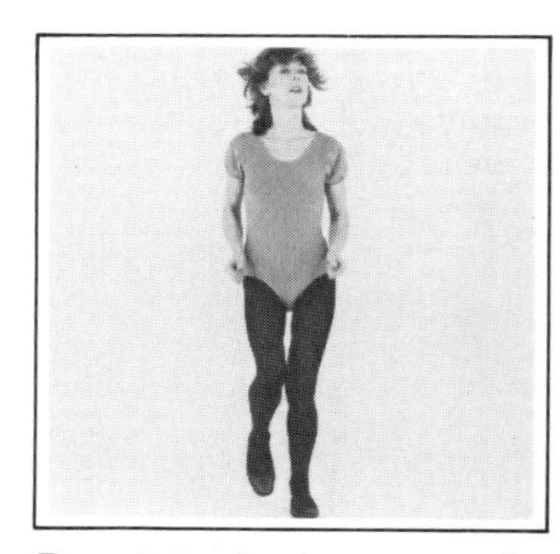

Do not stand or jump around to start execising.

9. Use as wide a base as possible. The wider the base the more stable the movement and the safer for the rest of the body. This applies whether doing office work, housework, lifting or carrying, etc.

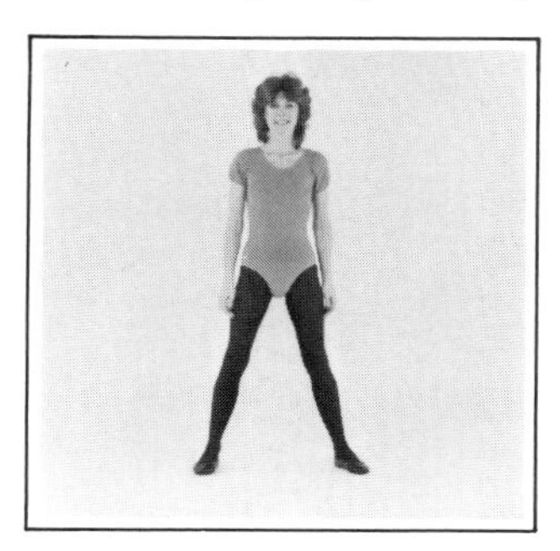

Do have a wide base if unfit – it makes you more mobile and more co-ordinated.

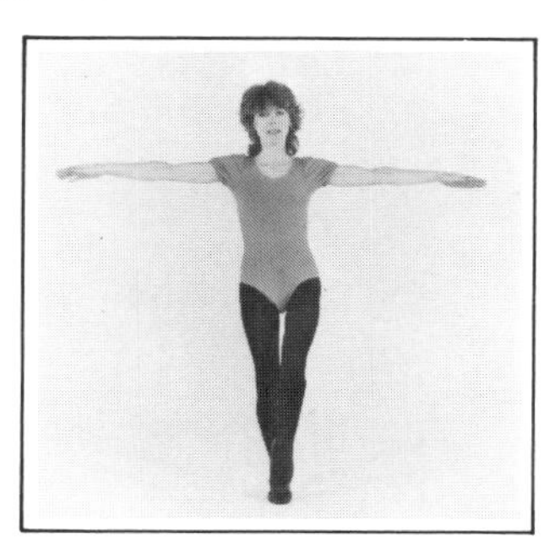

Do not have a narrow base if unfit – it makes you less mobile and co-ordinated.

10. Move your shoulders and arms before your head. There can be quite considerable stress and tension around the neck and it is safer to encourage the circulation by moving the big muscles of the shoulder girdle first before moving the neck (cervical) area which is the most vulnerable.

11. Move your head and neck slowly. When you move your head remember that the neck has many small joints and muscles which should be moved gently and carefully to prevent stress and strain.

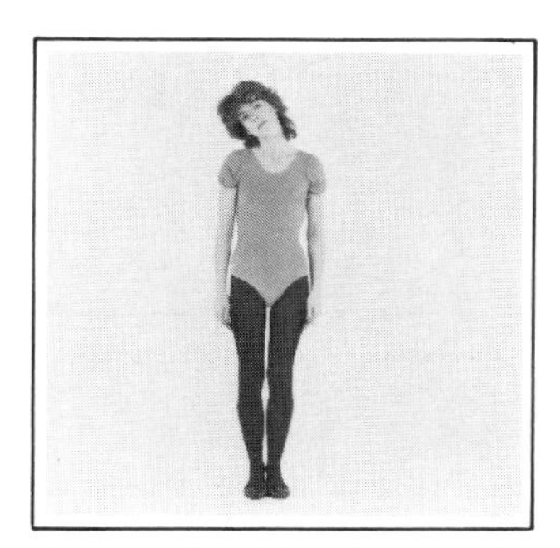

Do move head/neck slowly in all directions.

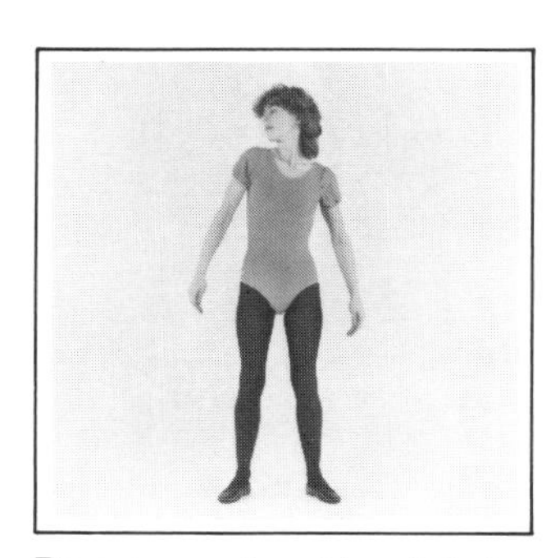

Do not move head/neck fast.

When Doing The Exercises

12. Exercise slowly and rhythmically. Rhythmical movements are safer and more beneficial than 'jerky' movements. Also a greater range can be achieved.

13. Bend knees in direction feet are facing. The knee joint can only move anatomically like a hinge so that the feet and knees must work together. If it moves in any other direction there must be a strain on the knee joint and possibly ankle too.

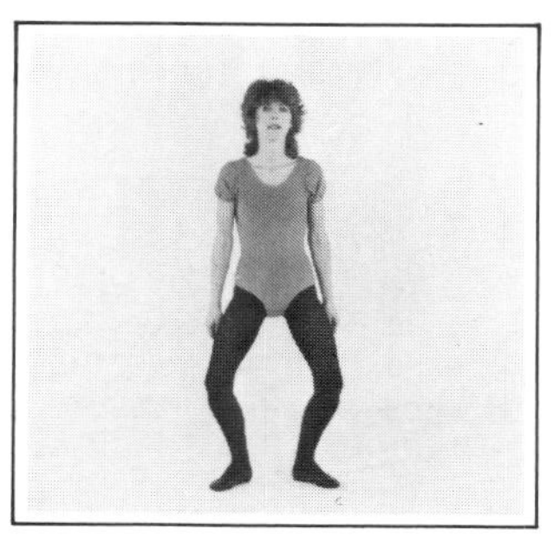

Do bend knees in direction feet are facing.

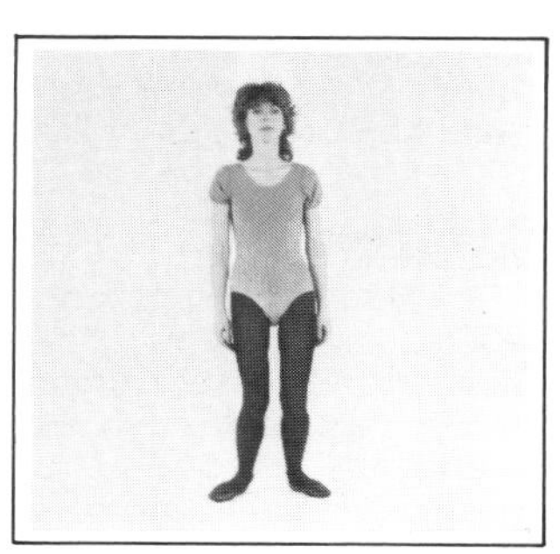

Do not bend knees in different direction to feet.

20 Guidelines to Exercising Well

14. Bend or relax knees. Most of us are not full time dancers with years and hours of exercise stretching the ligaments behind us! Be safe, always bend the knees when you reach towards your feet to prevent back injury. If you force a movement against a tight hamstring your back may give way.

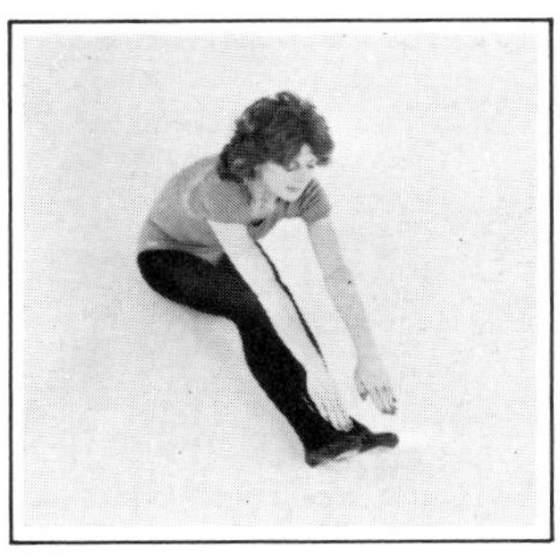

Do bend knees or relax knees if hamstrings are tight. **Do** go as far as is comfortable.

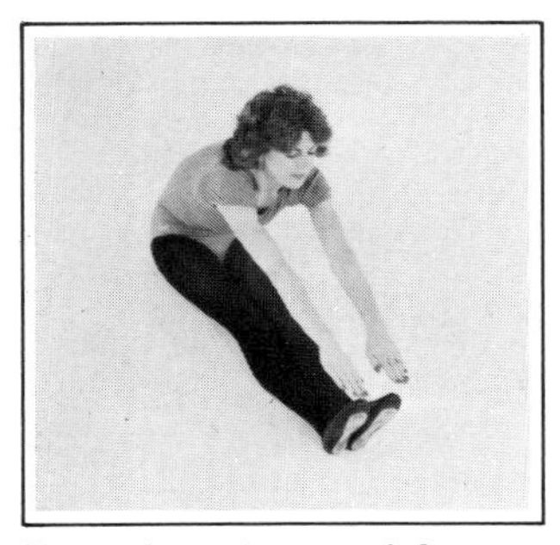

Do not keep legs straight, when hamstrings are pulling, i.e. tight. **Do not** force head onto knees.

15. Keep pelvis and knees facing front. If you swing the body from side to side when standing, either keep the knees and pelvis firm (e.g. facing the front) or move or pivot the feet to prevent any strain on the knees.

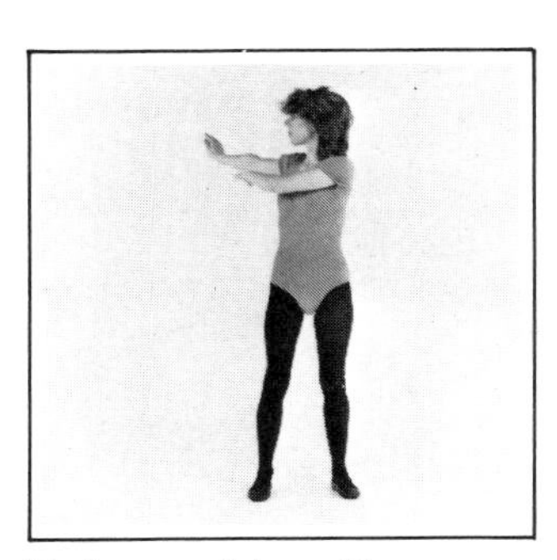

Do keep pelvis and knees firm and facing front, if feet are fixed.

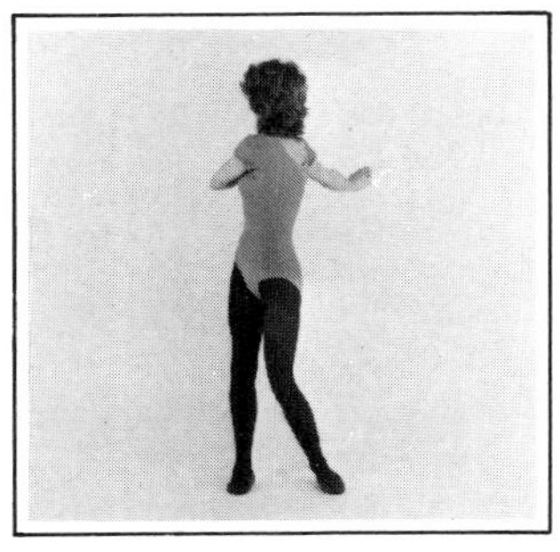

Do not twist knees and pelvis, if feet are fixed.

16. Always mobilise the spine from a supported starting position, e.g. sitting, prone kneeling or lying, you can then increase the range in safety and at your own pace. You can gently move it in all directions with the least discomfort and minimum aches and pains.

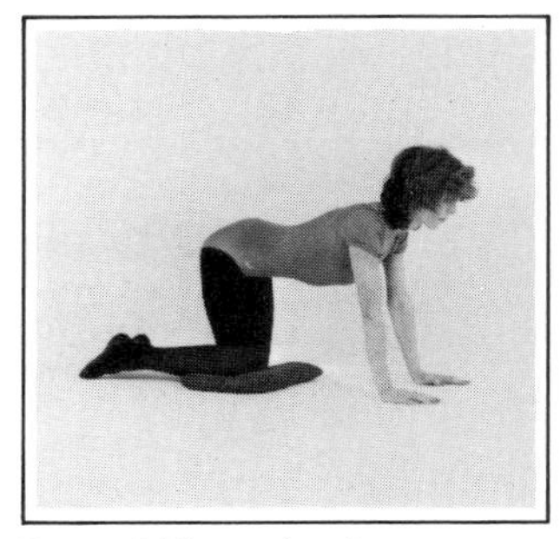

Do mobilise spine from supported starting position.

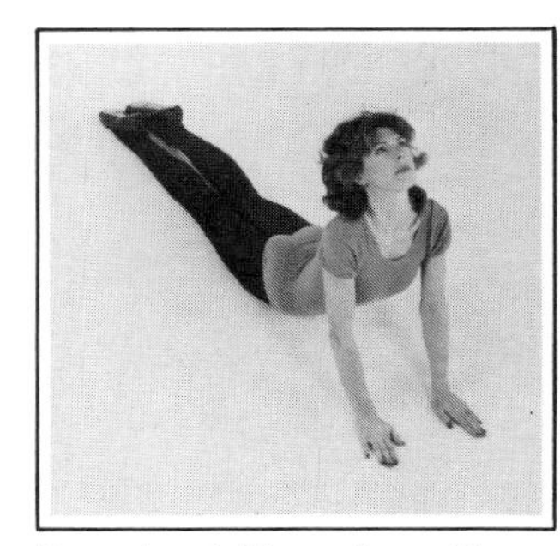

Do not mobilise spine with force or strength.

Take Extra Care With These Exercises:

17. Lower thighs parallel to floor when bending knees. The older the knees the easier it is to hurt the joint, especially with the body weight on top! Lower yourself as far as is comfortable and slowly return to standing. Never chance an injury whatever your age and forcing any exercise is dangerous.

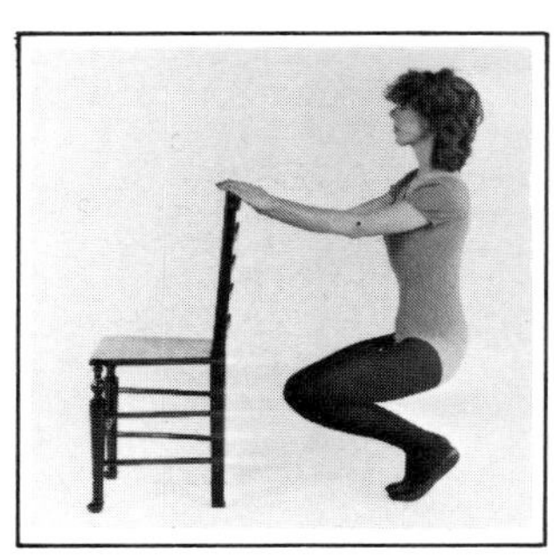

Do lower thighs only parallel to floor when bending knees slowly and return.

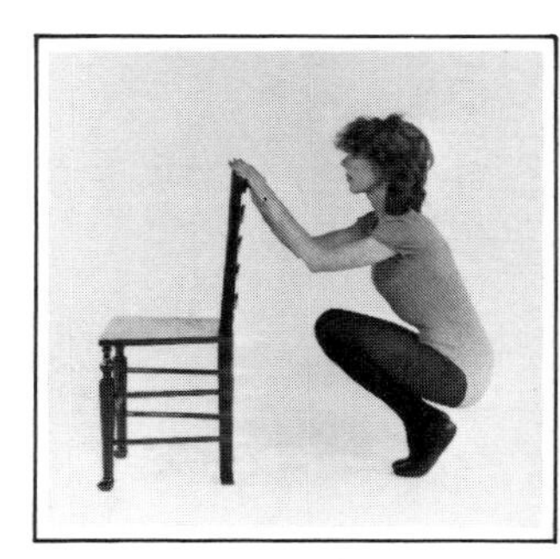

Do not over bend knees from standing or bounce.

18. Never lift both legs from the floor (from horizontal to vertical) at the same time. The hip flexors which lift the legs are attached to the lumbar spine. This means that the strain will be taken in this region especially if the abdominal muscles are not strong. Halve the strength by lifting one leg at a time.

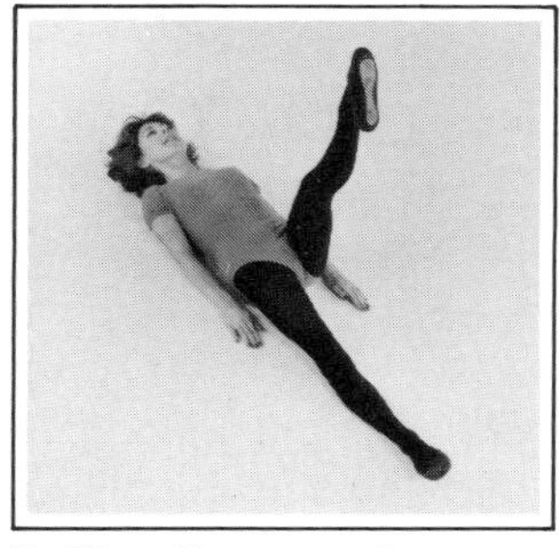

Do lift and lower one leg at a time from lying on your back.

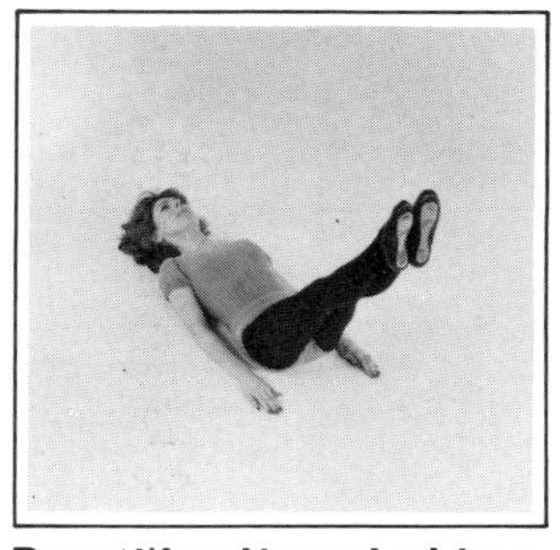

Do not lift and lower both legs at the same time.

19. Strengthen spine extensors without over arching back. It is not necessary in order to strengthen the back muscles to over arch the spine, or to lift the arms and legs at the same time which can be very heavy. This can compress the vertebrae and puts the lumbar region at risk.

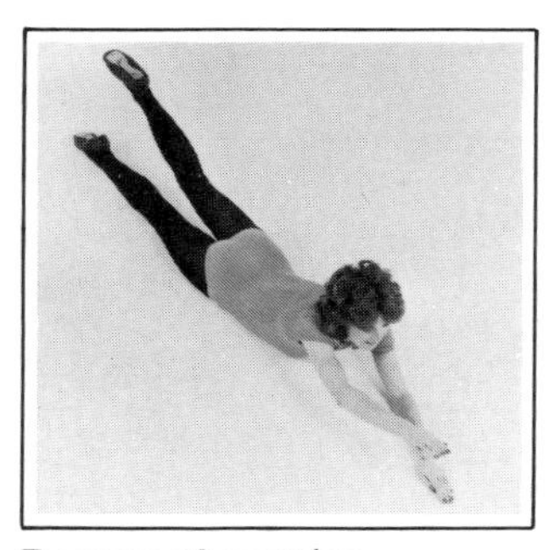

Do strengthen spine extensors without over arching back, raising one arm and one leg, or both arms, *or* both legs.

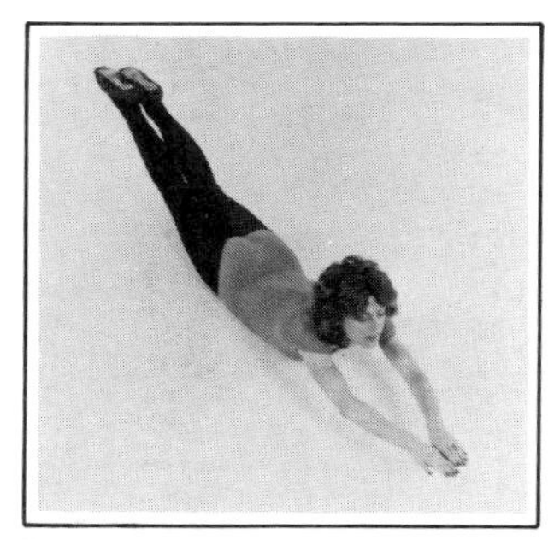

Do not over arch the spine, or lift both arms and legs at the same time or compress vertebrae.

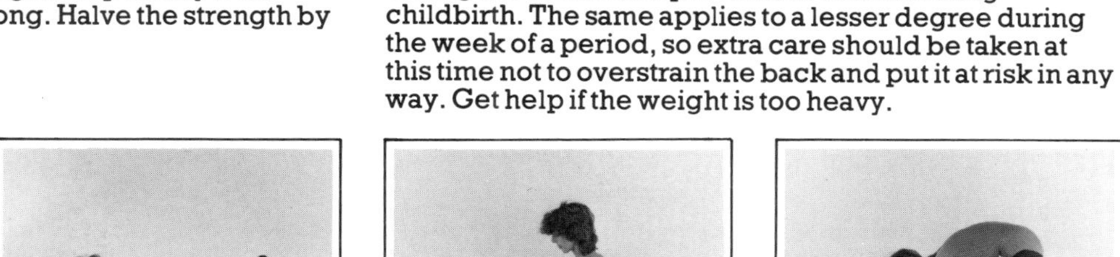

20. Keep back straight and bend knees when lifting. Because the hormones are preparing the body for childbirth, a woman's back is particularly vulnerable during the six months previous to and following childbirth. The same applies to a lesser degree during the week of a period, so extra care should be taken at this time not to overstrain the back and put it at risk in any way. Get help if the weight is too heavy.

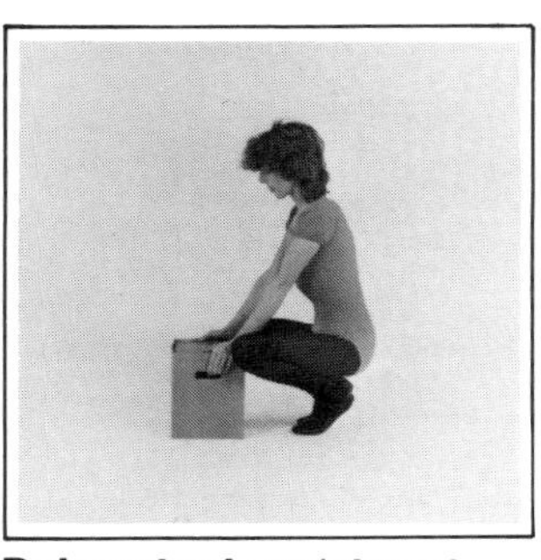

Do keep back straight and bend knees when lifting.

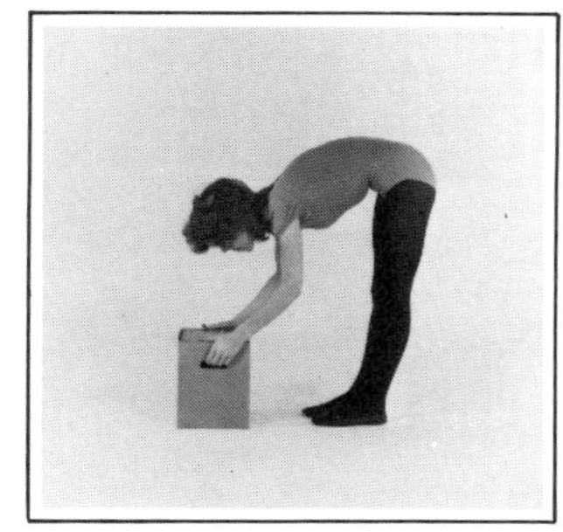

Do not round the back with the knees straight when lifting.

SAFETY

Safety Rules

Check your pulse rate. A slow pulse rate is characteristic of good Cardio Vascular Fitness (with longer rest periods for the heart, it is more efficient at pumping more blood per stroke, thus supplying more oxygen to the body). The average pulse rate is between 60-80 beats a minute.

Rest from exercising if you suffer from the following (and see your doctor if it persists):
- Rapid heart rate (i.e. 120 per minute, 5 minutes after exercise) extreme breathlessness, nausea or vomiting after exercise, prolonged fatigue.
- Side stitch (cramp in the diaphragm).
- Pain in the joints.
- Muscle strain.

Stop exercising and see your doctor if you experience:
- Dizziness, light-headedness, loss of co-ordination, confusion, cold sweat, glassy stare, pallor, blueness, fainting.
- Irregular or racing pulse, very slow pulse, fluttering, pumping or palpitations in the chest, pain or pressure in the arm or throat.
- Pain in the chest.

Never force your body when doing an exercise or do any jerky movements.

Listen and feel the messages from your body. There should be no pain involved in exercises.

After exercising you should feel pleasantly relaxed with more energy than before. If you feel tired, exhausted and fatigued after doing exercises you are overdoing it!

SECTION 2

EATING

THE SLIMNASTICS HEALTHY EATING PROGRAMME

Eating Well

Dieticians tell us that eating well means:

- Consuming a varied mixture of foods which provide all the nutrients the body needs in optimum proportions and at regular intervals.
- Making sure that the storing, preparation and cooking of food enhances the appeal to the senses but avoids any unnecessary loss of essential nutrients.
- Ensuring that the energy content of the food equates with but does not exceed the energy output needed by the individual.

This often differs considerably from one person to another.

We ordinary mortals have to put this theory into practice in our everyday lives.

In our Slimnastics Healthy Eating Programme we hope to prove that while concentrating on using a selection of foods which actively promote good health, and making sure we eat only the right quantities for our own metabolism, we can also make sure we enjoy it and produce food which:

Looks tantalising by using appetising colours and combinations.

Smells delicious by using aromas of spices and herbs, or newly cooked bread, ripe fruit, coffee.

Tastes mouth-watering and appealing by using natural flavours.

Feels comforting, enjoyable and satisfying.

Sounds crunchy by using fresh foods and methods of cooking which sizzle or bubble with anticipation.

Good food is one of the pleasures of life.

The Slimnastics Healthy Eating Programme

What is Food?

To understand which foods to choose and how they affect our health it will help to look at the composition of food and what happens to it inside our body. The human diet is usually made up from a mixture of foods which supplies the body with all the necessary nutrients. Most foods are themselves a mixture of nutrients – for example potatoes contain not only carbohydrates but are also a source of protein and other nutrients, and dairy foods have fat, protein and some vitamins and minerals. A *balanced diet contains a variety of foods* which include carbohydrates, proteins, fats, vitamins, minerals and water, and adds up to the right number of calories (i.e. energy input) for the individual metabolic rate and energy expenditure (i.e. output) so that no unused potential energy becomes stored as excess fat.

Carbohydrates include sugars, starches and dietary fibre. There are several types of sugars, the most common of which is sucrose which is quickly digested and absorbed by the body. *Starches* are more complex carbohydrates and they have to be broken down into simple sugars by the digestion before they can be absorbed into the body. The dietary fibre passes through the intestine without being absorbed.

For years it was considered to be a waste product but we now know that there is a whole family of plant fibres including cellulose, legnius (the woody part of plant cells) and gums and pectins each having its own unique properties. Some fibre absorbs water which gives food the bulk the bowel needs to make food pass along quickly; this may prevent unwanted matter from staying in contact with the bowel wall. Bacteria decompose some of the fibre and increase the bulk. The presence of some types of fibre prevents the re-absorption of cholesterol and bile acids. Fats, sugars, milk, eggs, fish, meat and alcoholic drinks contain no dietary fibre at all.

Proteins are made of groups of amino acids. Food proteins are broken down during digestion into these amino acids which are absorbed into the body. There are about 20 amino acids in the food we eat and in the body proteins. Eight of these must be provided from the diet and are called the essential amino acids. The others can be made by the body. Protein comes from both animal and vegetable sources such as meat, fish, eggs, milk and cheese, cereals and beans, peas, grain and nuts. For health we should try to increase the proportion of protein we eat from vegetable sources whilst reducing the proportion from animal sources.

Fats are the most concentrated source of energy and include a variety of chemical substances. Most fats contain mixtures of saturated and unsaturated fatty acids. Animal fats such as lard or suet have a relatively bigger proportion of saturated fatty acids. A large percentage of fat consumed by Western man comes from dairy products, especially milk. In nature milk is a food for babies only and has no place in the diet of adult animals. Dairy products are very high in saturated fats which have been proved to have a damaging effect on the adult body. For the sake of our health we need to severely diminish the amount we consume. Most oils from vegetable sources, such as corn oil, as well as fish fats contain relatively more unsaturated fatty acids. Processing can convert unsaturated fats to saturated fats as in the production of hard margarines. Some unsaturated fatty acids are essential to life because, like the essential amino acids, they are not synthesized by the body and can only be obtained from food. The body manufactures cholesterol as it needs it and the dietary intake is not therefore thought to have such importance. Certainly there is no need to consume saturated fats to make even more cholesterol.

Vitamins and Minerals. Food not only supplies the three nutrients from which energy can be obtained (carbohydrates, protein and fats), but also *Vitamins* which although only needed in small quantities are essential to the proper use of the other nutrients as well as our general health. Small quantities of about 20 *Minerals* are also necessary for the body.

Water is essential to maintain life. People can live for a much longer period without food than without water. We obtain water not only in drinks but also from foods such as fruit and vegetables.

Alcohol. Alcoholic drinks are a source chiefly of food energy although some contain very few minerals and some of the B vitamins. Although enjoyable they are not essential and if regularly taken may increase the energy intake above the body's needs (i.e. they are surprisingly high in calories) or may replace food leading to an inadequate nutrient intake. There is more about alcohol in Section 4.

Energy Needs

The amount of food a person needs varies with age, sex, size, activity, climate and the energy content of foods consumed. Every minute of the day people use energy to maintain body functions (such as heart beat, breathing, digestion and excretion) or as fuel for physical exercise. This is measured in kilocalories (calories); 1 kilocalorie is the heat needed to raise the temperature of 1 kilogram of water by 1 degree centigrade.

- Children have high calorie requirements in relation to their size because energy is also needed for growth. For the first ten years or so boys and girls of the same age have similar needs. Changes at puberty bring differences in growth rate, body size and activity patterns.
- Women need less energy than men because they weigh less and possess more body fat for insulation. This means they need less energy to keep warm.
- Even sedentary men need more than women doing comparable work. An average man uses up more energy daily just to keep alive.

How Much Is Enough and How Much Is Too Much?
With the right balance of food intake and energy output, the average person will maintain his proper weight. If the food intake is too much the excess will be stored as fat and the weight will increase; if the total food supply is too small to supply the body's needs, body protein will be used as a source of energy and muscle wasting will occur. No two people are alike and personal requirements for energy and nutrients will differ. Even in the individual they may change from day to day.

If we first concentrate on the most health-giving nutrients to supply our energy and then find we are still over our recommended weight, that is the time to cut down the calorie content of our daily intake. There is more detail on this in Section 4.

Ten Steps to Healthy Eating!

Eat More Fibre
This means eating more wholegrain cereals found in bread, pasta, rice, oats, etc.; a minimum of three portions of vegetables a day (one raw) including root vegetables (potatoes should be high on the list) and pulses, which also have a high proportion of protein as well as fibre

(these are the beans, peas, lentils, etc.); a minimum of 2/3 portions of fruit a day (fresh if possible).

You need to include all types of fibre as they have different beneficial functions.

The benefits you will achieve from eating more fibre will be to:

- Create a filling and 'satisfying' diet.
- Help avoid constipation.
- Reduce the possibility of diet-related illnesses such as appendicitis, cancer of the large bowel, diverticulitis, heart disease and gallstones.
- Remove the waste products from the body more quickly and easily.
- Possibly increase the amount of energy and fat passed in the stools.
- Decrease blood cholesterol.

Eat Less Fat

This means:

- Changing your cooking methods to grilling, baking, steaming.
- Spreading your fats such as butter and margarine very thinly.
- Choosing leaner, low-fat cuts of meat and low-fat offal (such as liver).
- Choosing chicken and fish more frequently.
- Substituting yoghurt for cream, and low-fat dressings for salad cream.
- Cutting out the 'visible' fats such as cream, fat on and in meat, all fried foods, only having a scraping of butter and margarine; cutting down 'invisible' fats found in cakes, biscuits, pastry, ice cream and such processed foods as pâtés, and tinned and 'manufactured' meats often found on the delicatessen counter.
- Cutting down on snack meals.
- Reducing the amount of cheese and nuts you eat which are high in fat.

The benefits you will achieve from eating less fats are definitely worth the effort!

- Fat is very high in calories and is very easy to overeat . . . if you cut the excess out you will control your weight.
- Fat helps to make us feel full so that cutting down leaves room for more beneficial foods, such as vegetables and fruits.
- High fat content in the diet is one of the factors in the development of heart disease, strokes, cancer, and obesity.
- Cutting down on fats will help reduce the level of cholesterol in the blood.

Eat No Extra Sugar

This means adding minimal sugar when cooking (try instead sweetening the more tart fruits with one of the sweeter kind – such as orange juice with rhubarb, dried sultanas with apples, etc.) The same applies to cereals and other dishes. Avoid foods containing sugar such as sweets, chocolates, puddings, biscuits, cakes, soft drinks and tinned foods, etc. You will find some dessert and breakfast ideas in Section 5. Always remember that *refined sugar* has no nutritional value except for providing energy.

The benefits you will achieve from cutting out the 'empty calories' of refined sugar are:

- A more interesting and better balanced diet. With less of your daily needs being fulfilled by these 'empty calories' you will be able to eat more bread, fresh fruit and vegetables including potatoes. These will add not only 'bulk' but also variation and good nutritional value as well.
- Easier weight control. After all, high energy = high calorie = probable overweight! You will find more about the high risk factors of obesity in Section 4.
- Less tooth decay. Dental surgeons have no doubt that refined sugar is the greatest single cause of dental caries especially when eaten frequently.
- More efficient use by the body of the food you eat. The rapid absorption of refined sugar from the gut may lead to the delay and decreased efficiency of the other food stuffs.

The latest Royal College of Physicians report on obesity suggests reducing sugar. The N.A.C.N.E. suggests that the sugar intake by the population of the U.K. should be reduced by 50%.

Watch Out for Salt

Our bodies need a small amount of dietary salt in order to function properly. At the moment we have on average approximately 11/12g per day whereas the World Health Organisation recommends only 5g each day and in this temperate climate we may even need less. It is now established that the blood pressure in a group of individuals is directly related to their salt content and there does exist an 'at risk' group of individuals who are susceptible to very high blood pressure (hypertension). As it is impossible to identify these individuals, everyone is advised to reduce their salt intake.

We obtain salt from three sources: it occurs naturally in food; it is added during processing, and we add it ourselves (this accounts for approximately 25%). We need to use natural flavourings whenever possible such as lemon juice, vinegars, herbs and spices, instead of seasoning with mainly salt.

We need to:

- Add no more than a pinch to cooking.
- Avoid putting the salt cellar on the table.
- Watch the salt content in processed and convenience foods. Read the ingredients list on the tins and packets especially those where you do not expect to see salt, such as breakfast cereals, crisps, peanuts, etc. – the taste tells all!
- Avoid artificially-made fizzy drinks.

The benefits of reducing your salt intake will be:

- A new awareness of the real taste of food.
- A decreased risk of high blood pressure and complications that can lead to strokes, heart attacks and kidney diseases.
- Experimenting with other forms of seasonings can be enjoyable.

Change Your Thoughts on Protein

Most people eat far more protein than is actually needed, and in particular proteins from animal sources which have the disadvantage of also being high in fats. Until recently prosperity has been equated with the amount of meat, milk, butter and cheese included in the diet. Even now these attitudes are reflected in advertising, and our reading material. The trouble is that most of us enjoy eating these foods and have got into the habit of thinking out our meals around them! We need a radical change in our priorities, for instance:

Think first of grains, pulses, and nuts! Change the proportion of protein from animal and vegetable sources. Increase the proportion from vegetable sources by reducing the amount of meat or dairy foods, and combining smaller quantities with a larger portion of vegetables in a dish. We give you some samples in Section 5. Use smaller portions of lean meat instead of larger portions of cheaper cuts of meat which have a high percentage of fat. Experiment by including more fish or game in your diet. Try vegetarian cookbooks for ways to cook pulses, grains and nuts.

The benefits you will achieve by eating more vegetable protein are:

- A much more varied, interesting and exciting diet.
- A less expensive shopping bill.
- A lowering of your calorie count which in turn helps control your weight.

The Slimnastics Healthy Eating Programme

- The prevention of the diseases mentioned above.
- The beneficial education of your children and their children so that they in turn live a longer, healthier life.

Care for Those 'Vital' Ingredients: Vitamins and Minerals
We all need adequate quantities of vitamins and minerals to keep healthy and well. The way to make sure of this is to eat a varied diet including cereals, low-fat dairy foods, fish, fruit and vegetables and perhaps some offal. Individual needs are variable and most of us have no need to worry. All of us need to make sure of a daily intake of Vitamin C because it is unable to be stored in the body and therefore needs to be replenished each day – it is found in raw fruits and vegetables but less so in cooked ones since it can be destroyed by overcooking or prolonged heat.

There are some groups of people who are vulnerable and particularly 'at risk' from a deficiency of vitamins and minerals. These are:

The housebound, the elderly, the very young and also those of Asian origin may need added supplements of Vitamin D. Vitamin D is called the sunshine vitamin because we manufacture it in our bodies from the rays of the sun; tablets need to be given under medical supervision.

Tobacco smokers. Smoking prevents efficient use of vitamin C, so smokers need to include extra in their diet.

Vegans. Vitamin B12 can be lacking in a vegan diet, so vegans need to be sure they get some from added sources.

Women, especially when pregnant, need to include the mineral iron in their diet. It is recommended that a food such as liver should be eaten by women every week.

Pregnant mothers need extra vitamins and minerals.

People who regularly drink alcohol. Alcohol alters the vitamin requirement of the body, especially those of the B group and so drinkers should supplement their diet with extra.

People on antibiotics. Antibiotics can influence the vitamins in the body especially vitamin B, and so additional vitamin B or multi-vitamin tablets should be taken.

Remember that:

- Unlike the soil, sea water is constant in minerals and its products are therefore reliable sources. Fish, shell fish and 'sea products' such as seaweed are high in minerals.
- Iron is much more easily absorbed in the form in which it occurs in animal foods than from vegetable sources. On the other hand if a food rich in vitamin C is eaten with an iron-containing food, more of the iron can be absorbed by the body, so that eating liver and onions together makes sure you fully benefit from these essential minerals.

For more information on vitamins and minerals in our diet, and where they are found, look at the lists in the appendix of this book.

Read the Labels
Labels on most pre-packed foods must include a complete list of ingredients. This will show in descending order of weight exactly what went into the food. Added water must be included as an ingredient if it makes up more than 5% of the weight of the finished product. Any food additives will be included in the ingredient list. Manufacturers are allowed to add certain substances to food, for colouring, flavouring, preserving or performing other functions. Food additives are usually listed by category names followed by the chemical name or serial number. A list of these can be found in the appendix.

Manufacturers want us to buy their products. It is in their interests to make sure it is as attractive, 'moreish', easy to prepare and within reach of our pockets, as possible. To this end they use colourings, seasonings (especially salt and sugar to which we have become accustomed and almost addicted), filling and satisfying fat, and delightful packaging to such an extent that we have confused these products with the real thing! We need to be very wary about the additives in our food. We now realise how detrimental the addition of salt and sugar is in our diet and some colouring agents (such as Tartrazine) and alternative sweeteners have also proved to be harmful to the health of some people.

Drink Alcohol for Pleasure Only!
Too many of us add the calories of alcohol to an already adequate diet (which causes added weight) or substitute the calories of the alcohol for food which will result in malnutrition. We do not need alcohol; it is not a necessary food!

For healthy living we need to limit our intake, in healthy eating alcohol has no place. It can however be an enhancer of good cooking.

- Read the page on alcohol under 'Life style'.

Eat Breakfast
Eating breakfast is good for your health. You need breakfast to aid concentration and keep you fit and alert during your working morning. Non-breakfast eaters are more liable to accidents and poor health. Food after our 'fast' during the night will help replace the dead cells, replenish the blood, balance the enzyme system and help rid the body of waste products. It is the fibre content of our breakfast which is the most vital; it is the fibre which collects the excess fat, cholesterol and unwanted matter and helps to ease their evacuation from the body. Everyone will benefit from some fibre in a meal as early to waking as possible.

- A quick economical meal of cereal or wholemeal toast will be more than adequate.
- Porridge or self-made muesli can be very good but read the cereal packets – some are very high in salt and sugar and if refined have lost much of the fibre.
- Try using skimmed milk or low-fat yoghurt instead of milk. Use added fruit for sweetening instead of sugar.
- Make sure the bread is wholemeal and again reduce the use of butter or margarine by either spreading thinly, or preferably using a low-fat spread. Cottage cheese, peanut butter, yeast extract (watch the salt), tomato, poached egg, mashed sardine or tuna fish (well drained) on toast are very good and do not need any butter or margarine added at all.
- By changing your diet in this way you should be including enough fibre. Only a very few people will need extra bran.

Balance the Energy
If you have been eating a high-fat, low-fibre diet and then changed to the pattern described above you are most likely not only to improve your general health but to very gradually balance your energy input with your energy output. It will take some time but you are likely to gradually achieve a reasonable weight for your height. However if you are already eating plenty of fibre, very little fat, no extra sugar, hardly any salt, a moderate amount of mixed animal and vegetable protein, limited alcohol, three meals a day and adequate vitamins and minerals, it is unlikely you have a weight problem! If you have, then you are probably simply eating too many calories. To carry too much excess weight is not only a health hazard in itself but carries with it the liability to being more prone to all diseases, it is a burden on your physical

posture and a depressant to your mental outlook. There is more about weight control in Section 4.

Taking Yourself in Hand

Step One *Find out what you are actually* eating. Most of us fool ourselves much of the time. If you write down completely honestly, your food intake for a week, the results will probably surprise you!

Step Two Start to plan a different way of eating, noting where you have been going wrong and the improvements you can make.

Step Three You eat what you buy . . . use the shopping list at the back of the book to give yourself a good start.

Step Four Experiment with different cooking methods and ideas. We give you plenty to try in the section on cooking.

Step Five Use your senses; try delicious herbs, heady spices, different colour combinations, lovely textures to improve your food.

Step Six Try a little self control! Look at the proportions on your plate, watch the quantities, count the calories if necessary or change the *way* you are eating!

Have a Bit of Courage!

Take it gradually step by step; eating differently can feel strange and disconcerting at first but it is a great adventure and very rewarding.

COOKING FOR HEALTH

A Reminder of the Principles

For healthy eating our objectives are:
- To eat more cereals, pulses, vegetables, fruit.
- To eat less fat.
- To exclude refined carbohydrates, e.g. white flour and sugar.
- To reduce salt to a minimum.

The recipes show you how to do this in practice.

Buying the Right Food You will eat what is available and in most cases this is what you buy. We have given you shopping lists of recommended foods to use at the back of this book.

Cooking by the Right Methods Cooking can improve the nutritional value of some foods such as grains by breaking down the indigestible cellulose envelopes enclosing the cells and making the contents more accessible to digestion and absorption. It also improves the tenderness and acceptability of meat and fish and can improve the digestibility of some vegetables. High temperatures are an important safeguard against food poisoning.

Careless and prolonged cooking can reduce or destroy the vitamin B and C content of fruits and vegetables. To preserve as much vitamin C as possible, fruits or vegetables should be cut with a sharp knife and plunged quickly into a little boiling water, the lid partly replaced to exclude most of the air and the vegetables cooked for the shortest possible time and never kept warm for long periods.

The good cook aims to produce food which has an attractive appearance and flavour (fresh ingredients such as herbs and spices for flavouring help here) and retain the natural colourings. These will not only stimulate the appetite and improve the appearance and acceptability of the foods but they also add, in most cases, valuable nutrients and properties in their own right. You will find a list of these to help you choose and select the most appropriate in the Appendices.

As you will be using minimum fat for this healthy eating programme it is vital not only to use the right method such as grilling, dry roasting or steaming, but also to have the most useful equipment.

Much of it can be improvised but it is a great help to have heavy non-stick pans, a wok, a vegetable steamer and a pressure cooker, and chicken and fish bricks can be invaluable too. A microwave is expensive but can be a quick and useful asset. You also need a strong pastry brush with which you can oil your pans lightly to avoid over-greasing them. Aluminium foil is good for making food parcels and can be used in place of the meat and fish bricks. Large oven dishes with covers are useful to retain all the food values and again a foil cover can be used instead of a lid if necessary. Kitchen paper is essential for soaking off excess fat or oil from tinned fish or sweated meat. Of course it goes without saying that a large pepper mill, several sharp knives of all sizes, wooden spoons and a rolling pin (to beat meat and fish as well as break nuts – not to roll out pastry) are necessities!

Preserving the Nutrients

Storing processing and preserving foods are part of our heritage. For many years vegetables have been pickled in vinegar, meat has been salted and cured, fruit has been preserved in sugar and food has been dried. Both for economic reasons and to meet the ever growing needs of an expanding world population a great deal of effort is devoted to increasing food supplies and to avoiding wastage of good food. The law permits specified preservatives to be added to many foodstuffs in order to safeguard them from microbiological spoilage. However, some preservatives are thought to be health hazards and it is widely recognised that the amounts consumed should be limited. We need to constantly question and be aware of the contents of the processed foods we buy and eat.

Today, food is increasingly being preserved by more modern means which avoid the addition of preservatives. These methods include sterilisation, canning, drying, dehydration and freezing. Sometimes the nutritional value of preserved food may be higher than that of fresh food which is of poor quality or has been badly prepared and cooked. For instance, good quality fruit and vegetables which are frozen immediately they are harvested, will probably be of greater nutritional value than similar produce which has been transported some distance to market and then to the retail shop only to find its way to the table after a considerable lapse of time.

Processing our Food has been found to be an insidious health risk in our modern world. Confusing 'white and pure' with 'goodness' led to the boom in the refining of our carbohydrates which in the case of sugar took out all the nutritional value and left only a highly concentrated source of energy that was easy to eat in excess of energy requirements and so tasty as to encourage us to develop cravings. Another good example is flour. The refining of flour not only removed the husk which provides us with essential fibre but also the 'germ' which contains the protein, mineral and vitamins.

In preparation too, vitamin C and some other vitamins can easily be destroyed in the factory or kitchen in several ways, such as by prolonged exposure to air after cutting up vegetables or fruit, by bruising or tearing with blunt knives or by soaking.

CEREALS

The three main forms of cereal used in cooking are flour, rice and pasta, but as usual, to make sure they add to our healthy way of eating these cereals must be used unrefined.

Wholemeal flour can be used in many recipes and for bread. Bread made with wholemeal flour can again be regarded as the 'staff of life'. As its name suggests, 'wholemeal' flour contains the whole grain including the bran and wheatgerm. This unrefined flour does not keep as well as white so it is best to buy only as much as you can use up in about one month. Keep the flour in the bag in which you buy it, remembering to mark it with the date of purchase. Keep it on a cool dry shelf or put it, still in the bag, inside a stoneware jar or other special floor jar. Never mix old with new flour. Yeast is the raising agent used in bread and is high in vitamin B content. It is a living organism and feeds on carbohydrates, e.g. starches and sugars which for your health's sake should always be unrefined. When it is mixed in dough and given the right conditions of warmth, moisture and food, it grows rapidly and gives off carbon dioxide which permeates the dough making it spongy in texture. Salt not only slows down the fermentation process but used in excess can kill the yeast. As in all cooking keep salt to the minimum.

Brown rice is cooked in the same way as white rice but it needs a longer cooking time. Boiling the rice takes about 25 minutes and by the absorption method it should be simmered for 45 minutes. Brown rice cooked in the oven needs about an hour.

The basis of pasta is hard durum wheat which grows particularly well in Italy. It comes in many shapes and sizes and is now available in wholegrain form. Pasta can be eaten with sauces of many kinds, including fish and meat, and also added to soups and broths to make a more substantial meal. It should be served when tender but still firm.

There are many cereals which have dropped out of popular use. Experiment, look for new recipes and read old recipes (the use of cereals used to be much more common). Keep an open mind. Add oatmeal to fish, cook vegetables with a topping of ground rice, put pearl barley in the stew. Look for different ways to put more cereals in your diet!

Remember if you are overweight some of the following recipes are high in calories and should be avoided until you reach the correct weight for your height as shown in the tables on page 50.

Wholemeal bread

1lb (450g) wholemeal flour
¾ tsp salt
¼ oz (7g) margarine
1 lvl tsp raw sugar
½ pt (285ml) warm water
½ oz (15g) fresh yeast
Wholemeal flour for sprinkling

Mix the flour and salt together on a working surface or in a large mixing bowl. Rub in the lard and make a well in the centre. Dissolve the sugar in the water and use 2 tablespoons of it to mix the yeast to a smooth paste. Add the rest of the water and pour into the well. Mix vigorously to blend in the flour and then knead for 5 minutes to make a smooth, elastic dough. Shape it into a ball and put in a warm greased bowl. Cover with a damp tea towel and set in a warm place to rise for 1 hour. Turn out the risen dough onto a working surface and knead out any air. Mould the dough into a ball and put it on a warmed and greased baking sheet. Cover with the tea towel and put back to rise in a warm place for 35 minutes, cutting a cross in it ½-inch (1.5cm) deep with a sharp blade after 20 minutes. Remove tea towel and bake in a pre-heated oven Gas Mark 8½ (460°F/235°C) for 35-40 minutes.

Oatmeal Bread

Replace 4oz of the wholemeal flour in the above recipe with 4oz (125g) fine oatmeal which adds a nutty taste and chewy texture.

Herb Scones

½ lb (225g) wholemeal flour
1 tsp baking powder
¼ tsp salt
1½/2oz (40g) low-fat margarine
¼ pt (140ml) skimmed milk
1oz (25g) chopped mixed herbs: chervil, dill, chives, parsley

Rub in everything together, add milk, roll out to ½" thick. Brush with skimmed milk, and bake for 12 minutes on Gas Mark 9 (475°F/240°C) on the top shelf.

Wholemeal Lunch Cake

1lb (450g) wholemeal flour
Pinch of salt
1½ lvl tsp baking powder
2 lvl tsp mixed spice
1 lvl tsp powdered cinnamon
6oz (175g) low-fat margarine or 3oz (75g) ordinary margarine
4oz (100g) raw brown sugar
3oz (75g) currants
3oz (75g) sultanas
2 eggs beaten
Approx. 10 tbsp skimmed milk

Line an 8-inch round cake tin. Combine flour, salt, baking powder and the spices in a basin. Rub in the fat then stir in the eggs. Add all other ingredients. Turn mixture into tin. Bake at oven centre, Gas Mark 4 (350°F/180°C) for 1¾ hours.

Wholefood Cake

14oz (400g) wholewheat or farmhouse flour
1 lvl tsp mixed spice
½ lvl tsp ground ginger
¼ lvl tsp salt
6oz (175g) margarine
6oz (175g) light brown sugar
1lb 2oz (500g) seedless raisins
2 lvl tbsp honey or black treacle
8 fl.oz carton natural yoghurt or buttermilk
1½ lvl tsp bicarb of soda
1 egg
Sprinkling of muscovado sugar

Grease and line 8-inch round cake tin. Put flour into a mixing bowl then sift in the mixed spice, ground ginger and salt; rub in the margarine; stir in the sugar and raisins. Put honey or treacle in saucepan with yoghurt or buttermilk and bicarb of soda and stir over a gentle heat until warm and frothy. Mix thoroughly into dry ingredients with egg. Spoon mixture into prepared tin, level surface and sprinkle with muscovado sugar. Bake just below centre of oven at Gas 4 (350°F/180°C) for one hour, reduce to Gas 3 (325°F/160°C) for further 45 to 60 minutes.

CEREALS

Muesli Bars

2oz (50g) glace cherries
2oz (50g) dried apricots
2 tbsp vegetable oil
4 tbsp real honey
3oz (75g) moist light brown sugar
5oz (150g) oat flakes
2oz (50g) sunflower seeds
1oz (25g) sesame seeds
1oz (25g) dessicated coconut or chopped hazel-nuts

Prepare a moderate oven Gas 4 (350°F/180°C). Lightly grease a shallow 7" x 11" (18cm x 28cm) oblong tin. Chop cherries and apricots. Measure oil and honey into medium sized saucepan, add sugar and oat flakes, sunflower seeds, sesame seeds and coconut. Mix well with spoon then knead together by hand to form firm mixture. Press into tin, bake at oven centre for 20/25 minutes until golden brown. Cut into 16 bars while still warm. N.B. These are high in calories and should be treats only!

Oat Crisps

2oz (50g) low-fat margarine
2oz (50g) raw brown sugar
1 egg
4oz (100g) crunchy oat cereal
3½ oz (90g) wholemeal flour
½ tsp baking powder
2 tsp instant coffee with a few drops hot water.

Cream together margarine and sugar until fluffy. Beat in egg. Add cereal, flour, and coffee essence, mix well and place teaspoonfuls, well spaced, on baking sheets. Chill for ½ hour. Bake in preheated oven Gas 4 (350°F/180°C) for 18 minutes until golden brown.

Bara Brith 'Welsh Tea Bread'

1lb (450g) wholemeal flour
4oz (100g) raw brown sugar
12oz (325g) mixed fruit
½ tsp mixed spice
1 dsp pure honey
2 eggs
1 cup cold tea
1 lvl tsp baking powder

Soak fruit in sugar and tea overnight. Next day, add rest of the ingredients and mix well together. Cook for approx. 1½ to 2 hours Gas 2 (375°F/190°C). Serve on its own or with a thin scraping of honey.

Yoghurt Bread

1lb (450g) wholemeal flour and bran
15.9oz (450g) carton yoghurt
1 tsp muscovado sugar
1 tsp baking powder

Combine all dry ingredients, mix together with yoghurt. Place in a 2lb bread tin. Bake for 1¼ hours at Gas Mark 2 (375°F/190°C). Serve with mashed banana and a squeeze of lemon juice.

Brown Rice with Herbs

2 medium leeks
1oz (25g) butter
1 tbsp oil
7oz (200g) brown rice
A few spring onions to taste
¾ pt (425ml) chicken stock
Sea salt and black pepper
1 tbsp chopped chives
1 tbsp chopped parsley
1 tbsp chopped dill
1 tbsp chopped basil
½ pt (300ml) natural yoghurt to serve

Trim, wash and slice leeks. Using an oiled pastry brush grease the bottom of a heavy saucepan and cook the sliced leeks slowly for 6/8 minutes in a little water. Wash and drain the rice and add it to the leeks. Stir for a minute or two. Add the sliced spring onions and pour on the heated chicken stock. Add pepper and herbs (if dried), cover the pan and simmer for 45 minutes stirring occasionally. By the end of the cooking time, the rice should be tender and the stock absorbed, if not, add a little more stock and cook for a further 5 minutes. If there is still some liquid left cook for a few more minutes uncovered. Add herbs now if using fresh. Serve with a bowl of yoghurt; it can be eaten on its own or used to accompany chicken or turkey cooked in an oven brick. Serves 4-6.

Noodle Savoury

1½ pt (850ml) chicken stock
8oz (225g) wholemeal noodles (ribbon type)
3oz (75g) streaky bacon, chopped
2oz (50g) sliced mushrooms
7oz (200g) can sweetcorn drained
2 tbsp low-fat plain yoghurt
2oz (50g) grated cheese

Simmer stock and noodles in a pan until all liquid has been absorbed. Fry bacon and mushrooms in non-stick pan for 2/3 minutes – pour off any fat. Add the noodles and the sweetcorn, stir in the yoghurt. Place in an ovenproof dish, sprinkle with cheese and brown under a hot grill. Serve at once; serve on its own, with a green salad or wholemeal bread. Serves 4-6.

Sesame Chicken with Spiced Rice

8 chicken breasts
6oz (175g) long grained brown rice
3oz (75g) wholemeal flour
pepper
½ oz (17g) powdered sesame seed or 1 lvl tbsp sesame seeds
½ pt (285ml) chicken stock
3 tbsp dry white wine
½ lvl tsp ground coriander
¼ lvl tsp ground ginger
Chilli powder

Cook the rice and when it is nearly ready, skin each chicken breast and roll the meat in the flour, black pepper and sesame seeds. Brush a heavy non-stick pan with vegetable oil and gently cook the chicken for 3 minutes on each side. Pour off any excess fat and then cover the chicken with the stock and wine. Cover pan with lid and cook gently for about 20-30 minutes until the chicken is cooked through. Strain the rice and then blend in the coriander, ginger, pinch of chilli powder and freshly milled black pepper. Arrange the chicken on top, keep warm. Boil the stock and wine very fast until it has reduced by about half. Pour over the dish and serve. Serve with a chicory and orange salad. Serves 4.

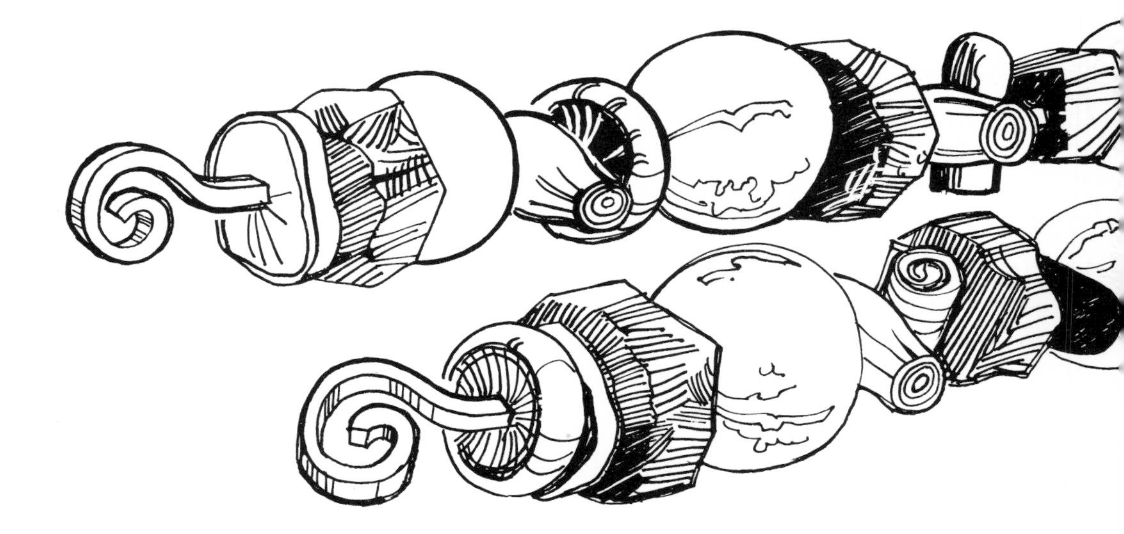

Greek Spiced Rice Ring with Kebabs

8oz (225g) long grained brown rice
Lemon juice
2 large ripe tomatoes
2 lvl dstsp finely chopped chives
2 lvl dstsp finely chopped parsley
8 green olives
½ tsp each dried basil, marjoram
1 red pepper
2 tbsp tarragon vinegar

Cook the rice with a teaspoon of lemon juice in the water until it is just tender. Drain and leave in a colander covered by a dry cloth to absorb the steam and keep the rice dry. Chop the tomatoes finely and combine with the chives, parsley, chopped green olives and dried herbs. Scald the pepper in boiling water, remove the stalk and seeds, cut into long strips, set 8 of them aside and chop remainder finely. Mix all of these into the warm rice, season with black pepper and lemon juice. Press this mixture firmly into a greased ring mould and leave to set in a cool place for at least 1 hour. Serve with kebabs which can include kidney, liver, onions and peppers. Serves 4-6.

Spaghetti with Lentils

14oz (400g) tin tomatoes
8oz (225g) cooked lentils
1 beef stock cube
1 onion peeled and finely diced

Combine all ingredients in a non-stick pan and cook until the onion is tender. Serve on a bed of wholemeal spaghetti cooked until soft but just firm. Serve with tomato and onion-ring salad. Serves 4-6.

Macaroni Mixture

3 rashers lean bacon (de-fatted and chopped)
1lb (450g) tomatoes (finely chopped)
1 green and 1 red pepper (blanched, de-seeded and chopped)
4oz (100g) sliced mushrooms
1 onion peeled and sliced
2 cloves garlic peeled and chopped
Pinch of tarragon, freshly milled pepper
Fresh parsley
Wholemeal macaroni as needed

In a wok (or non-stick frying pan) which has been sparingly greased, cook the bacon until the fat runs; pour off excess fat. Add the onion and garlic and cook until translucent, add the peppers and cook until tender, then the tomatoes and seasonings. Cook for a further 15 minutes. Pour over and mix with freshly cooked warm macaroni which is soft but just firm. Serve either on its own or with a Chinese Leaf salad. Serves 4-6.

Crispy Vegetarian Lasagne

10oz (275g) lasagne verde
6oz (175g) mature cheddar cheese
3 large onions peeled and diced
8oz (225g) mushrooms
2 medium courgettes diced
1 medium aubergine diced
2 small green peppers blanched and chopped
14oz (400g) tin tomatoes
2 cloves garlic, peeled and chopped
Pinch mixed herbs
Dash of Tabasco
Freshly milled black pepper
2 egg whites

Cook the onions in the sparingly greased non-stick pan until they are soft and transparent, add all the other vegetables and seasonings and cook for about 20 minutes. Cook the lasagne as directed on the packet. Lightly grease an ovenproof dish and grate the cheese. Put a layer of vegetable mixture on the bottom, then a layer of pasta and sprinkle with cheese, repeat ending with pasta. Top with stiffly beaten egg whites into which the remaining cheese has been folded. Bake in oven Gas 6 (400°F/200°C) for 30-40 minutes. Serve with a green salad or slice of wholemeal bread. Serves 4-6.

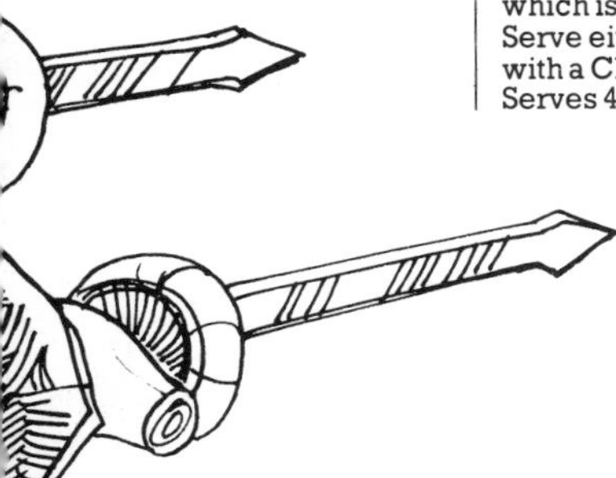

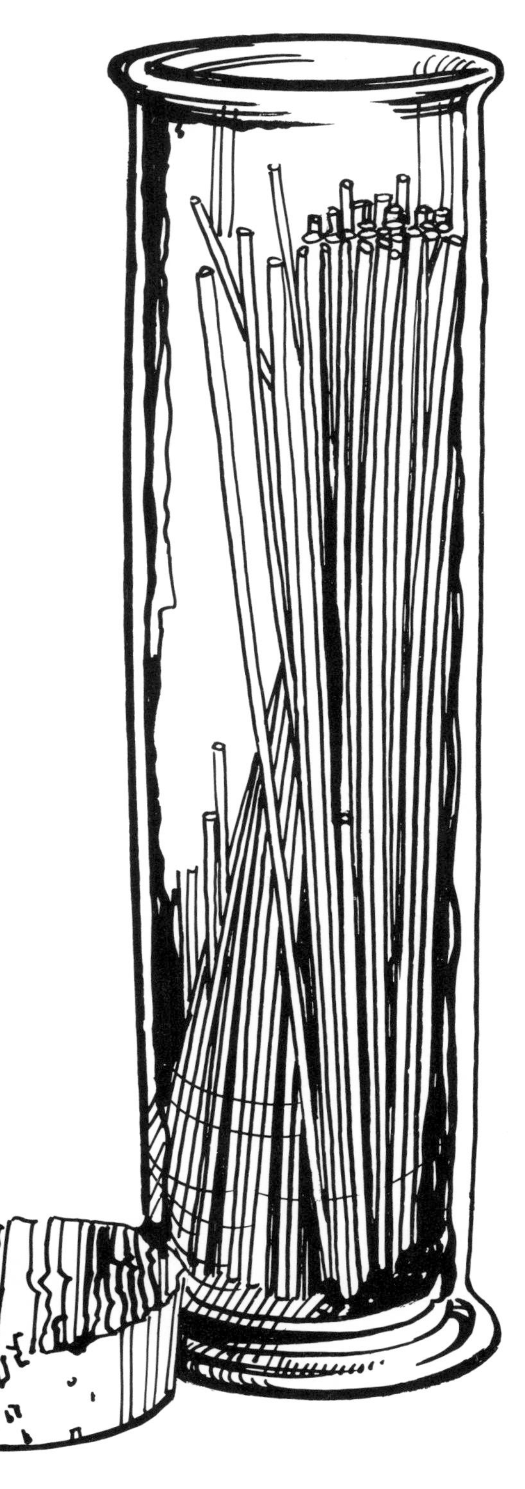

VEGETABLES AND PULSES

Freshness is all important when you are buying vegetables. The flavour of vegetables is at its best when they are young and firm and cooked as soon as possible after harvesting. Roots and tubers should be crisp and fairly free from soil; green vegetables should have no rotting leaves, they should look a good colour, crisp and fresh. There are so many different and sometimes unfamiliar vegetables on sale, there is a great deal of scope for producing interesting and tasty as well as nutritious dishes. All you need is a little courage and a sense of adventure.

Wash and rinse vegetables thoroughly but as quickly as possible in order not to destroy mineral salts and vitamins which are soluble in water. Only peel the root vegetables when absolutely necessary (such as when there are hard wooden patches or insect damage) as the most nutritious part of the vegetable lies just under the skin.

Do not despise the frozen vegetables, they are frozen within a few hours of picking and can be better quality and fresher than those which have been stored and damaged as well as polluted by dust and oil in their travels to the shops. Again vegetables which you have grown and picked yourself or even bought at source and then cooked or frozen are preferable. Do not forget the humble potato, it is much neglected and still for some, holds a 'fattening' image. It is an excellent way of adding bulk, stretching main dishes, as well as being nutritious.

As often as possible vegetables should be eaten raw but some root vegetables require cooking and there are times when a hot vegetable dish on its own can prove satisfying and enjoyable. We have chosen a variety of recipes using methods which retain the maximum nutrient value and fibre content of the ingredients as well as presenting different ideas and thoughts to spur you on to being more adventurous. None of these recipes are expensive or difficult. The quantities are for 4 to 6 people as this is the least extravagant way of cooking, if you do not need this amount and have not got a freezer, it is simple to quarter or halve the ingredients.

Pulses and beans are a very valuable and much neglected section of the vegetable selection. This is the general name given to the dried seeds such as green and yellow peas, haricot, butter and red beans and the green and yellow lentils. There are several more unusual ones which are also worth trying. These seeds are inexpensive and make a useful alternative to fresh vegetables, especially in winter. They also have a high protein content and make a valuable substitute in the diet for meat or fish. Try using them to stretch meat dishes or as a main dish on their own several times a week.

To prepare pulses pick over the seeds, discard any black or discoloured ones, and wash them under cold running water. Peas or beans should be placed in a large bowl and covered with cold water overnight. Lentils can be cooked without soaking. All kidney beans should be boiled at least 10 minutes to destroy the toxins. This is very important to remember if you are using a slow cooker.

Never add salt to pulses when cooking as it makes them tough. The cooking time varies depending on the type and age of the pulses and can be anything from 30 minutes to 2 hours. The cooking liquid can be set aside and used for making soups. We should endeavour to get used to using more pulses in our recipes instead of the animal protein; after all they are lower in fat content and high in roughage both of which are our aims!

Salt attracts moisture and if you put it on vegetables before cooking it draws out the juices. If you *need* to add some, apply sparingly after cooking.

Browned Toms

1lb (450g) tomatoes thickly sliced
1 large onion peeled and minced
2 rashers lean bacon (de-fatted and minced)
4 large slices of wholemeal bread made into crumbs
1 lvl tbsp chopped parsley
1½ lvl tsp chopped fresh (or dried) basil
Freshly milled black pepper

Mix the onions, bacon, breadcrumbs and seasonings together. Put half the mixture at the bottom of a greased, shallow, oven-proof dish. Cover this with a layer of tomatoes and season with pepper and continue with these layers until the ingredients are finished making sure that the top layer is the breadcrumb mixture. Bake at the top of a preheated oven Gas 5 (400°F/200°C) for 30-35 minutes until brown and bubbling. Serve with one of the salads from the following page. For a more substantial meal, cut out a hole in a small baking potato (1 per person), insert a lamb's kidney, replace a plug of potato and secure with a skewer. Bake alongside the tomatoes. Serves 4-6.

Dal Puri

8oz (225g) split yellow peas or lentils
saffron or turmeric
1 tbsp ground cummin
1 garlic clove
½ small onion, chopped
1lb wholewheat flour
½ tsp bicarb soda
salt & pepper

Pick and soak peas overnight, then boil with saffron or turmeric till fairly soft. Sweat cummin, garlic and onion together in a heavy pan brushed with oil over a low heat and add to peas. Grind well. A dry paste consistency is necessary so do not use too much liquid but watch to make sure it does not stick. Sift flour and bicarb of soda and add enough water to mix to a stiff dough. Form into balls the size of an orange, roll to ¼ inch thick, and put about 2/3 teaspoonfuls pea mixture in each circle. Fold over edges to cover the yellow mixture and roll out to ¼ inch thick again. Place on hot lightly greased griddle (or heavy-bottomed non-stick pan). Turn constantly and cook till brown and puffy – about 10 minutes. Serve with curry or tomato sauce. Serves 6.

Boston Baked Beans

1lb (500g) dried haricot beans
2 med onions chopped
1 tbsp black treacle or dark molasses
4 tbsp Worcestershire sauce
8oz (250g) bacon, chopped

Soak the beans for 12 hours. Drain and put into a saucepan with enough cold water to cover them by an inch. Simmer for ½ hour or until the beans are just tender. Drain. Put beans in deep casserole, add the other ingredients and enough boiling water to cover. Cover the casserole. Cook at Gas 4 (350°F/180°C) for 1½ hours. Uncover and cook for further 30 minutes. Alternatively the beans may be baked in a very slow oven for about 5 hours, uncovering them for the last hour. Add more water if the beans become dry. Serve with de-fatted gammon slices. Serves 6.

Soya Burgers

4oz (100g) soya beans (or 2oz plus 2oz kidney beans)
1pt (575ml) beef stock
2oz (50g) brown breadcrumbs
1oz (25g) wheatgerm
1 tsp chopped parsley (fresh or dried)
1 tsp chopped chives or grated onion
1 tsp mixed herbs
2 tsp tomato purée or ketchup (could use soya sauce)
black pepper
1 egg

Soak beans overnight. Discard the water the beans have been soaking in and cook in stock until soft; drain then mash or liquidise. Add other ingredients except for egg. Mix well and taste for correct seasoning. When correct bind with beaten egg. Form into burgers, coat in wholemeal flour and bake on lightly oiled griddle or heavy non-stick pan. Mixture may also be used for Scotch eggs. Serve with baked potatoes and green salad. Serves 4-6.

Lentil and Potato Pie

1lb (450g) potatoes, cooked and thickly sliced
3oz (75g) (dry weight) lentils, soaked overnight
1 large onion chopped and diced
8oz (225g) can tomatoes
2 tbsp tomato purée
1 tbsp Worcester sauce
2oz (50g) Cheddar cheese grated

Sweat the onion in a lightly-greased non-stick pan and add the tomatoes, tomato purée and Worcester sauce. Line the bottom of a lightly-greased oven-proof dish with potatoes, then arrange alternate layers of lentils and potatoes. Pour the tomato mixture on the top and sprinkle with cheese. Cook at Gas 5 (375°F/190°C) for 30-40 minutes and if necessary for a further 10 minutes at Gas Mark 3 (300°F/150°C). Serve with cooked tongue. Serves 4-6.

Vegetable Crumble

2 med onions
2 sticks celery
2 med carrots
2 med courgettes
½ small cabbage
½ small cauliflower
4oz (100g) mushrooms
4oz (100g) tinned tomatoes
4oz (100g) wholemeal breadcrumbs mixed with 2 tsp Parmesan cheese

Prepare vegetables by chopping or slicing, as appropriate, and gently sweat in a non-stick pan brushed with oil. Place in ovenproof dish and pour over tin of tomatoes. In a bowl mix the breadcrumbs, cheese and mustard. Place on top of vegetables and cook at Gas 6 (400°F/204°C) for 30 minutes until golden brown. Serve with baked or steamed fish or any meat. Serves 4-6.

Potato and Carrot Cake

8oz (250g) potatoes, scrubbed and sliced
8oz (250g) carrots, sliced
1 small onion chopped
2 tsp fresh sage, chopped or 1 tsp dried sage
3oz (75g) wholemeal self-raising flour
Black pepper and chives to garnish

Set oven to Gas 7 (425°F/220°C). Brush a non-stick pan with oil and sweat the onion until soft and translucent. Cover the potatoes and carrots with boiling water and simmer for 10-15 minutes, until tender. Drain and mash well. Add sage, onion, flour and seasoning. Mix well. Roll the dough into an 8-inch (20-cm) round on a lightly-floured surface. If the dough is too moist, add some more flour. Cut into 6 wedges and place these in the shape of a cake on an oiled baking sheet. Alternatively the cake may be left whole. Dust with flour. Bake on top shelf of oven for 30 minutes or until risen and golden brown. Serve hot (garnished with chives) with poached eggs and a green salad. Serves 6.

Cabbage Pie

2¾lb (1kg) onions, peeled and diced
7oz (200g) button mushrooms
5½oz (150g) carrots in small cubes
6/8 green cabbage leaves (de-ribbed and blanched)
Pinch of thyme and black pepper
2 eggs
2 dstspn skimmed milk

Brush the bottom of a non-stick pan with an oiled pastry brush. Sweat the diced carrots for five minutes and then add the onions. Continue to cook slowly for a further 15 minutes until they are soft and the onions translucent. Add the mushrooms and the seasonings and cook for further 10 minutes. Meanwhile drain and pat dry the cabbage leaves with a cloth and line a greased cake tin 6-inch (16-cm) with them. Leave enough hanging over the sides to fold over the top and completely enclose the filling. Beat the eggs lightly into the skimmed milk, take the vegetables off the heat and mix the two together. Fill the cake tin with the filling and enclose it with the cabbage leaves. Cover with aluminium foil, put the tin in a baking dish or bainmarie which has been partially filled with water. Bake in oven Gas 7 (425°F/220°C) for 50 minutes. Take the pie out of the oven and allow to stand for 10 minutes. Turn it out onto a round serving dish. Serve with tomato sauce which has been made with a tin of tomatoes which has been drained, mashed and heated, seasoned with garlic, oregano and freshly milled black pepper. Serve with slices of liver that have been gently poached in the tomato sauce and placed on top of the pie. Serves 4-6.

Spinach Soufflé

4 shallots peeled and finely chopped
1lb (450g) spinach, washed and very finely chopped
Freshly ground pepper
5.29oz (150g) carton of low-fat plain yoghurt
2 egg yolks beaten
3 tsp parmesan cheese
¼ tsp Cayenne pepper
5 egg whites whisked

Brush the bottom of a non-stick pan with oil and cook with shallots over a low heat until soft (about 5 minutes). Add the spinach, cover the pan and cook in its own juices until tender (roughly a further 5 minutes). Pour off the liquid and season with pepper. Mix the egg yolks and yoghurt, Parmesan cheese and Cayenne thoroughly and add to the vegetables when cooled. Fold in the egg whites and pour into a greased 1½-pint (850-ml) soufflé dish. Place in centre of pre-heated oven Gas 5 (375°F/190°C) for 30-40 minutes until puffy and golden brown on the outside and still runny on the inside. Serve immediately with a fresh green salad. Serves 4-6.

Turnips with Orange Sauce

Juice of 2 oranges
1½lb (700g) young turnips, peeled and quartered
½ pt (285ml) chicken stock
Coarsely grated rind of 1 orange
Freshly ground black pepper

Put the orange juice in a saucepan with turnip quarters. Add enough stock to just cover the turnips. Cover and simmer gently for about 30 minutes or until tender. Drain the turnips in a colander, reserving the liquid and put them in a warmed serving dish. Put the cooking liquid in a small saucepan and boil rapidly until reduced by half. Sprinkle the grated orange rind and freshly ground pepper over the turnips and pour the sauce on top. Serve with baked white fish. Serves 4-6.

Parsnips with Walnuts

2lb (900g) parsnips cut into matchsticks
1lb (450g) tomatoes thinly sliced
Juice of 1 orange
Pinch of oregano
Freshly ground black pepper
2oz (50g) chopped walnuts

Put the pieces of parsnip into a vegetable steamer or wire colander and place over a pan containing a few inches of water. Cover pan tightly and bring to boil. Steam gently until parsnips are tender (about 15-20 minutes). Put half the parsnips at the bottom of a greased oven-proof dish. Cover with a layer of tomato slices, pour on half the orange juice, some pepper and a pinch of oregano, repeat and top with the walnuts. Put in a preheated oven Gas 5 (375°F/190°C) and cook for 20 minutes. Serve with any of the dishes in the meat section e.g. Veal in Almond Sauce, Rabbit with Mustard etc., and add a green vegetable. Serves 4-6.

Polish Cabbage

2lb (900g) red cabbage, shredded
1 large sliced onion
5 tbsp wine vinegar
1 large eating apple diced
2oz (50g) sultanas
½ tsp of nutmeg/cinnamon/caraway or allspice if desired

Boil the cabbage in water for 10 minutes. Drain, reserving 1½ pints (850ml) cabbage water. Sweat the onion in a non-stick pan which has been brushed with oil, until soft and translucent. Add 1 pint (570ml) cabbage water to make a sauce. Mix together the cabbage, sauce, vinegar, apples and sultanas and spices and cook over low heat for at least 1½ hours, stirring occasionally to prevent sticking. More cabbage water may be added if the mixture becomes too thick. Add freshly milled black pepper. Serve with ham, tongue or oily fish. Serves 6.

SALADS

We should eat some fresh raw fruit and vegetables every day and salads are the perfect interesting way to serve them. Combining the right textures, colours, tastes and shapes is an art and a matter for experimentation, trial and error. Do not regard a salad as only 'rabbit food'! You can use a host of different ingredients with dressings and herbs that enhance the flavour. The only stipulation is that the materials used should be at their very best. This need not be expensive as you will be using the fruits and vegetables in season. We have not stated the quantities below as often that is a matter for individual taste. We have only given you ideas, to stimulate you into thoughts of your own. Enjoy the experience; it is good for your health and pocket, and will satisfy and sharpen your palate too.

- Apples, celery, walnuts, lemon juice.
- Avocados sliced, lettuce leaves, white wine vinegar, black pepper, oregano.
- Bean sprouts, cress, cucumber, onions, baked almonds, pepper, mint, lemon juice.
- Beetroot (freshly cooked) thinly sliced, low-fat yoghurt and horseradish to taste.
- Brown rice (cooked but not cooled), oranges, celery, yellow pepper, sultanas, sunflower seeds or peanuts, aduki beans (cooked), orange juice and white wine vinegar, chives.
- Carrots (sliced thinly at the last moment), mandarins, orange and lemon juice, mint.
- Cauliflower (blanched), with white wine vinegar, chives and grilled almonds.
- Chicory cut into long strips with orange or tangerine slices, orange juice, chives.
- Courgettes, onions and different peppers, diced and blanched with garlic, parsley and lemon juice.
- Cucumber diced with low-fat yoghurt and mint.
- Cucumber thinly sliced and alternated with halved strawberries, orange juice and black pepper.
- Dandelion leaves (very young) or spinach, crispy bacon, garlic, white wine vinegar, black pepper.
- Leeks thinly sliced, and blanched with sliced bananas marinated in lemon juice.
- Mushrooms thickly sliced with lemon juice and low-fat plain yoghurt.
- Pineapple (fresh and cut into chunks), lettuce, celery, oranges, cucumber thinly sliced, lemon juice, pinch of ginger.
- Pulses and beans cooked (of all shades and shapes) mixed with gherkins.
- Red, green and yellow peppers diced and mixed with diced tomatoes, garlic and pepper.
- Red cabbage shredded, pickled beetroot, french beans, oregano, black pepper.
- Spinach, spring onions, mushrooms, hard boiled eggs, garlic and orange juice.
- Tomatoes and onions thinly sliced with chives and basil.
- Watercress and orange slices.

SOUPS

Soups are warming, appetising, filling and full of good ingredients. They can be a starter to a meal or a whole meal in themselves. We have given a few recipes here but obviously there are many more. The points to note are that very little fat is used or needed (indeed if you have made your own stock it is important to let it cool long enough for any fat to float to the top so that it can be removed), that the vegetables are (with the exception of the onions and garlic) never peeled; that potatoes, cereals (like pearl barley and wholemeal bread), egg yolks and yoghurt can all be used as thickening instead of flour, and that the garnishes are added at the last moment so that they retain their nutrients. With such excellent food thermos flasks so easily available, soup can easily be taken to work or on a journey. To complete a meal accompany it with a piece of wholemeal bread. *Note:* We have supposed that you are the owner of a liquidiser or blender but the use of this machine is purely for ease and speed. In fact a better consistency is achieved by painstakingly pressing the bulk through a sieve or passing through a food mill. We have also given the quantities for 4-6 servings as it is easier and more economical to cook in these amounts. A freezer can be invaluable as well as a saving to a small household as soups freeze well and can be kept in single or double portions as desired. Otherwise halve or quarter the quantities to be used. Soup does not necessarily have to be liquidised, it can be very interesting if the ingredients are simply chopped in even-sized pieces.

Fisherman's Chowder

12oz (325g) potatoes (sliced but not peeled)
14oz (400g) tin tomatoes
12oz (325g) whiting fillets or other white fish mixed, diced
2oz (50g) peas
2oz (50g) sweetcorn
Black pepper, lemon juice and parsley to taste
2oz (50g) prawns for garnish (optional)

Cook the potatoes with the tinned tomatoes until they are soft, blend in the liquidiser until smooth, return to the pan with the fish, vegetables and seasonings and simmer for another 10-15 minutes. Just before serving stir in the lemon juice and garnish each bowl with the parsley and prawns. Be careful not to overcook this soup or the delicate texture of the fish will be spoilt and become rubbery.
Serves 4-6.

Vegetable Soup with Chervil

8oz (225g) carrots
2pts (1.1l) chicken stock
8oz (225g) turnips
12oz (350g) courgettes
Sea salt and black pepper
4 tbsp plain yoghurt
2 tbsp chopped chervil

Peel carrots, cut them in thick slices and put in saucepan with the stock. Bring to the boil and simmer for 5 minutes. Add turnips, peeled and cut into chunks, cook for a further 10 minutes. Add the courgettes, unpeeled and cut into thick chunks, cook for 12-15 minutes until all vegetables are soft. Push through a coarse food mill or purée very briefly in a blender. Reheat and add freshly milled pepper. Stir in yoghurt and the chopped chervil and serve. (When chervil is not available parsley can be substituted.)

Artichoke Soup

1lb (450g) large Jerusalem artichokes
1 small onion diced and peeled
1 clove garlic, peeled and finely chopped
1 stick celery, washed trimmed and chopped
2pts (1.1l) chicken stock
White pepper
5.29oz (150g) carton yoghurt (plain low-fat)
Garnish: Toasted almond flakes

Wash the artichokes, put them in a pan of fast boiling water and boil for five minutes. Drain and let them stand. Brush the bottom of a non-stick pan with oil and add the onion, garlic and celery. Sweat over a low heat for 10-15 minutes until the onion is soft and transparent. Add the chopped artichokes and continue stirring over a low heat for 2 minutes. Add the stock and seasonings and simmer for about 30 minutes until the artichokes are completely tender. Drain and reserve stock. Blend the vegetables and return to the pan together with the stock and bring to the boil again. Just before serving stir a tablespoonful of yoghurt into each bowlful and garnish with the almonds. Serves 4-6.

Danish Soup

4oz (100g) dried yellow split peas
2oz (50g) pearl barley
2pts (1.1l) stock (chicken or beef)
1 small onion peeled and diced
Freshly ground black pepper
A bay leaf
2 tbsp tomato purée
A dash of Tabasco Sauce
Garnish: Chopped parsley

Put the peas and barley together in a large basin, cover well with water and leave to soak overnight. Next day drain them, and blanch in boiling water for 2 minutes. Drain well. Then put the peas and barley in a large, heavy-based saucepan with the stock and onion. Season with the pepper and bay leaf and bring to the boil. Simmer for 1 hour. Mix in the tomato purée and continue to simmer for another 30 minutes until the peas and barley are absolutely tender. Remove the bay leaf and add Tabasco Sauce to taste. Blend in a liquidiser. If the soup is too thick add some more stock. Serve garnished with parsley. Serves 4-6.

Lebanese Cucumber Soup (Chilled)

1 large or 2 small cucumbers
14oz (400g) carton yoghurt
1 clove garlic
2 tbsp tarragon vinegar
2 tbsp finely chopped mint
Black pepper to taste
Garnish: Sprigs of mint

Wash and dry the cucumber. Do not peel but grate it coarsely into a bowl. Stir in the yoghurt. Peel and crush the garlic and together with the vinegar add to the cucumber. Season to taste with freshly ground black pepper and stir in chopped mint. Chill the soup in the refrigerator for at least 1 hour. Garnish with sprigs of mint. Serves 4-6.

Leek Soup

2 med onions peeled and diced
8oz (225g) leeks, washed, trimmed and thinly sliced
2½oz (65g) wholemeal bread, diced
2pts (1.1l) chicken stock
Freshly ground black pepper
Garnish: Crumbled crispy bacon

Brush the bottom of a non-stick pan with oil. Sweat the onions and leeks over a low heat for 10-15 minutes, stirring occasionally until soft and transparent. Add the bread and stock and bring to boil. Season with pepper, cover and simmer for 30 minutes. Liquidise the soup in a blender and return to a clean pan to reheat. Garnish each serving with crumbled crispy bacon which has been baked in the oven on a wire tray to lose as much fat as possible. Serves 4-6.

Lettuce Soup

8oz (200g) lettuce leaves
1 small onion
2pts (1.1l) chicken stock
Black pepper, grated nutmeg and fresh orange juice
1 egg yolk
5.29oz (150g) carton plain low-fat yoghurt

Wash the lettuce leaves thoroughly and plunge them into boiling water, allow the water to come to the boil again and then drain and rinse under cold running water. Chop the leaves; peel and dice the onion. Brush the bottom of a non-stick pan with oil, gently sweat the onion and then add the shredded lettuce (saving a little for garnish) and seasonings. Pour on the stock and bring to the boil. Just before serving take off the heat and beat in the egg yolk. Serves 4-6.

Pea Soup

3 rashers gammon bacon (diced)
1 large onion, peeled and diced
2 med carrots, chopped
1lb (450g) dried peas, soaked overnight in cold water to cover
4pts (2.3l) chicken stock
Black pepper and 1 tsp Worcestershire sauce
Garnish: Chopped parsley

Put the bacon in a large, heavy-based saucepan and cook over a gentle heat until the fat runs out. Pour this off. Add the onion and carrot and sweat gently until soft. Drain the soaked peas and add to the pan with the stock. Bring to the boil and add the seasonings, cover and simmer for about 2 hours until the peas are mushy. Blend in the liquidiser, adjust the seasonings and re-heat. Garnish with parsley. Serves 4-6.

Tomato and Carrot Soup

1 small onion peeled and diced
2 cloves garlic peeled and finely chopped
6oz (175g) carrots diced
1lb (450g) tomatoes, roughly chopped
1 small eating apple cored and chopped
2pts (1.1l) chicken stock
Bouquet garni of thyme, marjoram and 3 bay leaves
Freshly ground black pepper
Garnish: chopped chives

Brush the bottom of a non-stick pan with oil. Put in the onion and garlic and sweat over a low heat until soft and transparent. Add the carrot and stir over the heat until soft. Add the tomatoes, apple, bouquet garni and stock, season and bring back to the boil. Cover and simmer for 45 minutes. Remove and discard the bouquet garni and blend the soup in the liquidiser. Return to clean pan, heat through and adjust seasoning. Garnish with chopped chives or if in season marigold petals.

Chicken, Egg and Mushroom Soup

(Cooked in a wok)

4oz (100g) raw chicken
2 eggs
6 chinese mushrooms
4oz (100g) watercress
1 slice ginger root
¾pt (425ml) stock
½ stock cube (chicken)
¼ tsp pepper
1½ tbsp port (if desired)
Lemon juice

Soak mushrooms in lemon juice for 30 minutes. Cut chicken into thin slices. Cut the mushrooms into thin slices. Add 4 tablespoons of mushroom juice to the stock. Wash watercress and separate if necessary. Brush oil over the wok and gently cook chicken strips, add mushrooms and stir for 1 minute. Pour in stock and bring to boil. Add stock cube and ginger and simmer for 3 minutes. Add chopped watercress and rest of ingredients and stir for 2 minutes. Pour beaten eggs into soup and fold in gently. Serves 4-6.

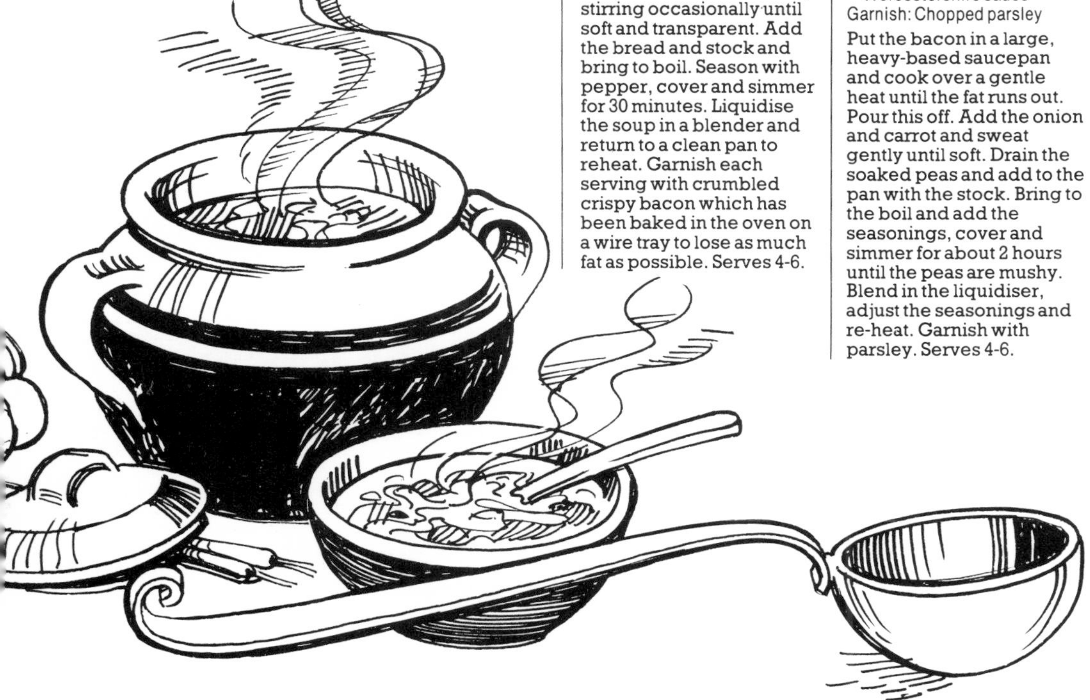

FISH

Fish provides, pound for pound, slightly more protein than meat. Oily fish contains mainly unsaturated fat which also carries vitamins A and D which gives an added nutritional value. White fish are low in fat, more easily digested than oily fish and are less calories. Both white fish and oily fish can be bought fresh but if you live inland they're probably more 'fresh' if you buy them frozen, than if you buy them from a fishmongers.

Fresh fish has a firm texture with a shiny, smooth skin. Avoid fish that is flabby and limp with dry, dull skin that dents when you touch it. Check that the eyes are bright and full, not sunken and opaque. The gills should be bright red, not pale. There should only be a slightly fishy smell. Do not buy fish that smells strongly, with any scent similar to ammonia, as this indicates decay. River or oily sea fish go off more quickly than other types and must be looked at more closely.

To eat fish at its best, cook it the day you buy it. Never overcook fish, it will toughen the flesh and destroy the flavour. Test for readiness by inserting a skewer. It is cooked when the flesh separates easily from the bone or when a soft white liquid similar to curd oozes out of it.

Britain is a fishing country and yet we eat comparatively little fish. It is an excellent food and perhaps the delicious recipes that follow will help persuade you to eat more.

Beryl's Tuna Tomatoes

2 large tomatoes or 4 smaller ones
7oz (200g) tin of tuna fish
2 tbsp plain yoghurt
4 spring onions diced
Lemon juice
Garnish: Lettuce and chopped chives

Cut tomatoes in half and scoop out the flesh. Discard the seeds and mix the flesh with the drained mashed tuna, diced onions and lemon juice. Stir in the yoghurt and put the mixture into the tomato shells. Serve garnished with chives on a bed of lettuce. Serve as a starter or as a supper dish with wholemeal bread. Serves 2-4.

Crispy Fish Pie

12oz (325g) courgettes thinly sliced
2 med red eating apples, cored and thinly sliced
1 large onion sliced
½ tsp dried sage
1½ lb (675g) rock salmon cut into small chunks
Black pepper
1 heaped tsp dry mustard
2oz (50g) fresh wholemeal breadcrumbs

Heat oven to Gas 5 (375°F/190°C). Layer a greased oven proof dish with courgettes, apple and onion. Sprinkle with sage, cover and bake for 30 minutes. Add the fish and seasonings. Mix the dry mustard with breadcrumbs and sprinkle over the fish. Bake for a further 25 minutes. Serves 4-6.

Stuffed Marrow Rings

1 med marrow peeled, de-seeded and cut into rings
15oz (425g) tin pilchards in tomato sauce
Pinch of paprika
1 egg white
Pinch of Parmesan cheese

Put the marrow rings in a vegetable steamer and place over a saucepan of hot water. Steam until tender. Mash the pilchards in a bowl and add a pinch of paprika. Carefully transfer the marrow rings to a lightly oiled shallow ovenproof dish. Fill with the pilchard mixture. Top with beaten egg white into which has been folded a pinch of Parmesan cheese. Place in the top of a previously heated oven Gas Mark 7 (425°F/220°C) until golden brown (about 10-15 minutes). Serve with Browned Toms or some of the other vegetable dishes in the previous section. Serves 4-6.

Seafood Hot Pot

1½ lb (675g) cod or haddock fillets
1lb (480g) potatoes, thickly sliced (but not peeled) and blanched
2 cloves garlic, crushed
2 large onions, finely sliced
4oz (100g) shelled prawns plus several whole prawns to garnish
3oz (75g) mushrooms
8oz (225g) tomatoes roughly chopped (or one large tin drained)
1oz (25g) wholemeal flour
½ pt (285ml) dry white wine or water
½ lemon squeezed
Fresh parsley and lemon slices to garnish

Set oven to Gas 4 (350°F/180°C). Sweat the onions in a lightly-greased non-stick pan and add garlic until soft and translucent. Stir in flour. Add the wine (or water) and lemon juice and stir well. Remove from heat. Cut fish into chunks. Slice mushrooms if large, otherwise leave whole. Mix all ingredients except the prawns together and put into a casserole. Cover and bake for 1 hour. Stir in the prawns until warmed through. Garnish with parsley, lemon slices and whole prawns. Serves 4-6.

Herring & Oatmeal Bakes

2lb (900g) whole fresh herring
Wholemeal flour for dusting
2 eggs beaten
Black pepper
4oz (125g) porridge oats
½ tsp dry mustard powder
2 oranges sliced
Parsley to garnish

Clean and remove heads from the herrings. Split along the belly, open the fish and place, skin uppermost on a board. Press firmly along the back of the fish, turn over and remove the backbone. Wash and dry on kitchen paper. Cut the fillets into 2-inch (5-cm) strips and dust with flour. Dip in egg seasoned with pepper and coat in oats mixed with mustard. Bake in preset oven Gas 7 (425°F/220°C) until golden brown (about 15 minutes). Serve piping hot on a plate covered with orange slices. Garnish with parsley.

N.B. Oily fish such as herrings, mackerel, sprats, etc., do not need any added fat when they are baked in the oven. All these fish are suitable for this dish. Serve with puréed vegetables such as parsnip or swede.

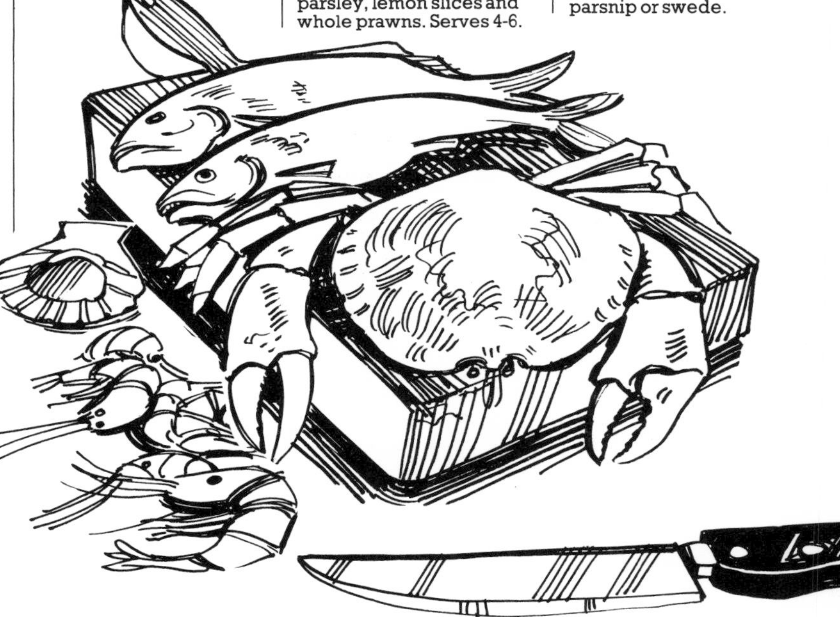

Salmon Mousse

1lb (500g) salmon, fresh (cooked and flaked), or tinned.
1 tbsp capers
1 tbsp gelatine
¼ pt (140ml) skimmed milk
2.5fl.oz (70ml) water
2.5fl.oz (70ml) red wine vinegar
1 tsp salt
1 tsp dry mustard
Watercress and cucumber to garnish

Soften the gelatine in the water in a bowl. Place the bowl over boiling water and stir until the gelatine dissolves. Add the remaining ingredients and stir. Put the mixture into a lightly oiled ring mould (or individual moulds) and chill until firm (about 6 hours). Remove from the mould and garnish with cucumber slices and watercress. Serve with cucumber and strawberry salad sprinkled with a good measure of black pepper.

Carnival Crab Salad

1 large or 2 med cooked crabs (enough to give 12oz (325g) meat) – tinned is equally successful
3oz (75g) cooked pasta shells
3oz (75g) cucumber diced
3 tomatoes peeled and diced
1 lettuce washed and shredded
Black pepper
Lemon juice
¼ pt (140ml) low-fat plain yoghurt and lemon juice
Watercress and paprika pepper

Remove the meat from the crab, dice and mix together with the pasta shells, cucumber and tomatoes. Season with black pepper and lemon juice. Arrange the shredded lettuce in the base of glass dishes and divide the crab mixture between the dishes. Top each with yoghurt mixed with lemon juice. Serve as a starter garnished with watercress and a sprinkling of paprika pepper. Serves 4-6.

Fish Parcels

This is an easy, clean and nutritious way to serve individual fish. It is also a way to pre-prepare fish for a dinner party especially for a number of people. The whole fish is wrapped in a parcel of foil and served unwrapped in its parcel direct to the table. The fish may be filled with appropriate stuffings for instance:

Trout Filled with a tsp each of lemon juice and vermouth with black pepper and dill or fennel.

Plaice Fillets can be wrapped around a piece of avocado pear with chopped tomatoes with lemon juice and a hint of basil.

Mackerel May be filled with horseradish mixed with yoghurt.

Red mullet With a filling of anchovies and red port.

Cod With a covering of mustard mixed into yoghurt.

Scallops With a teaspoon each of orange juice, white wine and a pinch of ground mace.

The parcels can be made in advance and stored for a few hours in a refrigerator. They should be cooked in a pre-heated oven at Gas 7 (425°F/220°C) for 15 to 20 minutes depending on the thickness of the fish.

Bigger fish can be baked with these fillings or flavourings in a fish brick. In this case the temperature should be lower and the timing longer. The tastes however will be excellent. Serve one fish per person with brown rice or new potatoes (unscraped), peas and a green salad.

MEAT

We are omnivorous animals and have got used to eating a lot of meat. To improve our health we would be wise to begin to radically change our attitudes and habits. We need to eat smaller quantities of meat, especially the red meats such as beef, lamb and mutton, and eat white meat (found in poultry, veal and rabbit or fish) more often. The main problem is of course the fat. Meat is mottled with saturated fat particularly in mature animals. The cheap cuts of the meat tend to be higher in fat. The more expensive cuts are the tender, more protected and less fatty or bony parts. We therefore need to think in terms of buying the more expensive cuts but in smaller quantities than before. This means we have got to think of how we can stretch small portions of meat with cereals or vegetables to make appetising dishes.

Fat gives meat its juiciness and much of its flavour. So to prevent dishes being dry and dull we must either marinate the meat pieces (soak for several hours in red or white wine, cider, beer or stock with herbs and then drain before cooking), or cook with other foods and moisture to not only add taste and bulk but also the missing nutrients such as carbohydrates, fibre, vitamins and minerals to meals.

We have endeavoured in the accompanying recipes to give you some ideas how this can be achieved. You can adapt many other recipes in this way: reduce the meat, add more vegetables or cereals, and eliminate any extra fat. It should not be necessary to add more fat as most cuts contain sufficient. You can cook your meat in a covered dish which will retain the moisture.

As meat contains no fibre, include fibre-containing dishes in the rest of the meal. Kebabs are a good example of this: alternate small meat or offal slices with pieces of vegetables, (which have been blanched or which cook easily) and serve with brown rice. Kidneys can be stuffed into holes made in potatoes and then baked. Small steaks (beef or lamb) can be grilled or oven baked and then eaten with one of the vegetable dishes. If you do roast joints raise them above their own fat on a wire tray and when carving remember to slice thinly! Each piece of meat should be treasured. It should now be thought of for high days and holidays not as a normal rule.

MEAT

Veal with Almond Sauce

3oz (75g) blanched almonds toasted
1 clove garlic peeled and chopped
1lb veal (450g) lean veal, beaten thin and sliced in long thin strips and rolled in wholemeal flour
½ pt (285ml) chicken stock
2 tbsp sherry
3oz (75g) pimento-stuffed olives
6oz (175g) sliced mushrooms
8oz (225g) cooked wholewheat noodles
Garnish: Orange slices and parsley

Break the almonds into small pieces by crushing them on a board with a rolling pin. Brush the wok (or heavy non-stick pan) with oil and sweat the garlic gently. Add the floured strips of meat and gently brown. Pour in the stock and sherry, cover and cook for 15 minutes. Add the almonds to the wok, increase the heat and stir the dish while the liquid reduces. Add the olives and the mushrooms, cook for a further 2 minutes and pour over the cooked noodles to serve. Garnish with the orange slices and parsley. Serves 4-6.

Chilli con Carne

2 large onions peeled and diced
1lb (450g) carrots, diced
2 cloves of garlic, peeled and chopped
12oz (325g) lean beef cut into small cubes
8oz (225g) tin of tomatoes
3oz (75g) tomato purée
1 bay leaf
1 tsp each cummin, oregano, cayenne
2 tbsp chilli powder
2fl.oz (50ml) beef stock
14oz (400g) red kidney beans already cooked

Brush the bottom of a heavy non-stick pan with oil. Sweat the onions, carrots and garlic until soft, add the meat cubes and when browned add all the other ingredients (except the beans). Cover and simmer for 1 hour. Add the beans and cook for a further 30 minutes. Serve with brown rice.
Serves 4-6.

Wheatgerm and Lamb Casserole

1oz (25g) margarine
1oz (25g) wholemeal flour
½ pt (285ml) skimmed milk
½ pt (285ml) stock
8 black pepper corns
½ tsp paprika
2 tsp Worcestershire sauce
1lb (450g) fresh peas, weighed after shelling
2 med leeks, trimmed and finely chopped (use whole of leek including green parts)
1 celery stalk trimmed and chopped finely
¼ tsp each dried sage and basil
1lb (450g) cooked lean lamb diced and de-fatted
2 tbsp chopped fresh parsley
5 tbsp wheatgerm
2oz (50g) Edam cheese grated

In medium-sized flame-proof casserole, melt the margarine over a moderate heat. Remove the casserole from the heat and, with a wooden spoon, stir in the flour to make a smooth paste. Gradually add the skimmed milk, stirring constantly and being careful to avoid lumps. Add the crushed peppercorns, paprika and Worcestershire sauce. Return the casserole to the heat, gradually add the stock and cook, stirring constantly for 2 to 3 minutes or until the sauce is thick and smooth. Reduce the heat to low and add the peas, leeks, celery, basil and sage. Cook, stirring constantly for 5 minutes. Add the lamb, reduce the heat to very low and simmer for a further 15 minutes. Do not allow the mixture to boil. Stir for a further 15 minutes. Do not allow the mixture to boil. Stir in the parsley and 2 tablespoons of the wheatgerm. Preheat the grill to high. Remove the casserole from the heat. Sprinkle the remaining wheatgerm and the cheese over the mixture. Place the casserole under the grill until the cheese has melted and is bubbling and golden brown. Remove the casserole from the heat and serve immediately, straight from the casserole. Serve with wholemeal macaroni or noodles. Serves 4-6.

Tangy Chicken in a Brick

1 roasting chicken
2lb (900g) gooseberries, fresh or frozen
Mint leaves to taste
15.9oz (450g) low-fat plain yoghurt
Freshly milled black pepper

If the chicken is frozen make sure it is completely defrosted. Put it into the chicken brick (or large oven-proof dish). Completely surround with the gooseberries and put the mint leaves on the breast. Cook at Gas 4 (350°F/180°C) for 1 hour or until the chicken is thoroughly cooked. Strain off the excess liquid and reserve for stock (removing fat when cooled). Press the gooseberries through a sieve to remove the pips and when cool blend with the mint leaves and yoghurt, season with pepper. Pour the sauce over the chicken to serve. Serve with brown rice and salad. Serves 4-6.

Herby Chicken in a Brick

1 roasting chicken or chicken pieces
8oz (225g) plain cottage cheese
2 tbsp low-fat plain yoghurt
1 tbsp lemon juice
1 tbsp each fresh chopped parsley, tarragon, chives
Freshly milled black pepper

Carefully lift the skin up from the chicken breast or pieces. Mix the cottage cheese, yoghurt, lemon juice and herbs together in a bowl. Pack this under the skin of the chicken. Put in the chicken brick (or very large oven-proof dish with lid), breast upwards. Place the lemon skin (half from which the juice was squeezed) inside the chicken. Bake in the preheated oven Gas 4 (350°F/180°C) for 1 hour or until the chicken is completely cooked. Pour off excess liquid and retain for stock (removing fat when cooled). Serve with baked potatoes and salad. Serves 4-6.

Moussaka

12oz (340g) lean lamb cut into small cubes
2 large peeled and diced onions
2 garlic cloves peeled and chopped
3 med aubergines diced
2 tbsp tomato purée
3fl.oz (75ml) red or white wine or small tin of tomatoes
1 tsp ground cinnamon
1 tbsp chopped fresh parsley
Freshly milled black pepper
Topping: 1 egg separated
5.29oz (150g) carton low-fat plain yoghurt
2oz (50g) cheddar cheese grated
Small dash made-up mustard

For this dish you need two lightly-oiled heavy non-stick pans. In one gently sweat the garlic, onions and small cubes of meat. In the other put the aubergines to sweat slowly. When the meat is browned add the wine, tomato purée and seasonings. Cover the pan and simmer gently. Pour the excess fluid off the aubergines, cover this with a layer of the meat mixture and continue in this way leaving at least ½" at the top of the dish. Cover and put in the centre of preheated oven Gas 4 (350°F/180°C) to bake for 1 hour. When the dish is done, stir the egg yolk into the yoghurt, whisk the egg white until stiff and fold into the yoghurt mixture with the cheese and dash of made-up mustard. Take the lid off the moussaka, pour over the topping, increase the oven temperature to Gas 7 (425°F/220°C) for 5 minutes or until golden brown. Serve with green noodles. Serves 4-6.

Fruity Turkey Parcels

6 turkey breasts or large slices of turkey
8oz (225g) mixed dried fruit (apricots, prunes, etc.)
2fl.oz (50ml) red wine or port (water if preferred)
Black pepper

Soak the dried fruit in the red wine or port overnight. Beat the turkey breasts until they are thin and flat. Put each piece on aluminium foil. Chop the dried fruit into small pieces and put some in the middle of each piece of meat. Fold the breasts over and make into parcels with the foil making sure they are completely sealed. Bake in a preheated oven Gas 6 (400°F/200°C) for ½ hour. Serve with brown rice and green vegetables. Serves 6.

Chicken Pot Roast with Herbs

3½lb (1.6kg) chicken, preferably fresh
Black pepper
Lemon juice
3-4 sprigs dried fennel
1 sprig rosemary
2 bay leaves
1 bunch thyme
2 sage leaves
1 bulb garlic
¼ pt (140ml) dry red wine or tin of tomatoes

Season inside of chicken with lemon juice and pepper. Place in a chicken brick in which the herbs have been scattered. Split the garlic bulb but do not peel then place round the chicken. Season and pour over red wine. Cover and cook for 1½ hours, Gas 6 (400°F/200°C). Serve with minted new potatoes that have been blanched and then baked with the chicken, and a salad.
Serves 4-6.

Rabbit with Mustard

1lb (450g) rabbit pieces
1lb (450g) mixed root vegetables (carrots, turnips, parsnips, etc.) peeled and chopped
2 large onions peeled and chopped
3 tbsp Dijon mustard
¼ tsp thyme
6fl.oz (175ml) white wine or de-fatted chicken stock
Freshly ground black pepper

Brush the bottom of a heavy non-stick pan with oil and gently sweat the onions and the mixed root vegetables. When the vegetables are soft and the onions transparent add the rabbit pieces and cook until they are just brown. Pour off the excess fluid and add the mustard and other seasonings. Mix well and then pour on the wine. Bring to the boil and continue to stir for 2 minutes. Transfer the ingredients to an oven-proof casserole and bake in a preheated oven Gas 5 (375°F/190°C) for 1 hour until the rabbit is tender. Serve with baked potatoes. Serves 4-6.

Casserole of Hearts

4 lamb or 2 calf hearts
Juice of a lemon and an orange
8oz (225g) onions
2 med cooking apples (or eating apples)
2 rounded tbsp wholemeal flour
Black pepper
2 bay leaves
¼ pt (140ml) cider or pure apple juice
1 lvl tsp coriander seeds
2 thin slices unpeeled lemon

Cut the hearts into slices, about ½-inch thick, and remove all fat, gristle and blood vessels. Put the slices in a basin with the lemon juice and leave to marinate for 30 minutes. Meanwhile peel and slice the onions and core and slice the apples. Dry the heart slices and coat them with the flour. Grease a heavy non-stick pan and sweat the onions gently until they are transparent, add the heart slices and brown them gently. Put a layer of onions and heart slices in an oven proof dish, cover with apple slices then a layer of heart and so on until dish is full. Pour in the cider, lemon juice, orange juice, seasonings and top with lemon slices. Cover the dish and cook in a preheated oven Gas 2 (300°F/150°C) for 1 hour or until the hearts are tender. Serve with baked potatoes, puréed parsnips or swedes. Serves 4-6.

Turkish Chicken with Rice

4lb (1.8kg) roasting chicken
10oz (250g) natural yoghurt
½ lvl tsp ground ginger
½ lvl tsp turmeric
½ lvl tsp ground cumin seed
¼ lvl tsp chilli powder
1 lvl tsp garam masala (omit rather than substitute)
1 lvl tsp salt
1 clove garlic
2 bay leaves
1 tbsp tomato purée
grated rind of 1 lemon
ground black pepper
A little paprika
1 lemon cut into six wedges
½lb brown rice (uncooked weight)

Joint the chicken. Put yoghurt into a large bowl and mix in ground ginger, turmeric, ground cumin seed, chilli powder and garam masala, crushed garlic, salt, bay leaves, tomato purée, lemon rind and ground black pepper. Add the chicken pieces and leave to become well saturated with the yoghurt and spices. Make sure all pieces are well coated, cover and leave for at least 24 hours in a cool place. Remove bay leaves. Place chicken on a wire rack in roasting tin. Spoon over remaining yoghurt mixture and sprinkle paprika on top. Bake Gas 4 (350°F/180°C) for about 1½ hours until chicken is tender and crisp, and golden brown in colour. Meanwhile cook the rice. Place on dish and put chicken joints on this and decorate with wedges of lemon. Serve with green salad. Serves 4-6.

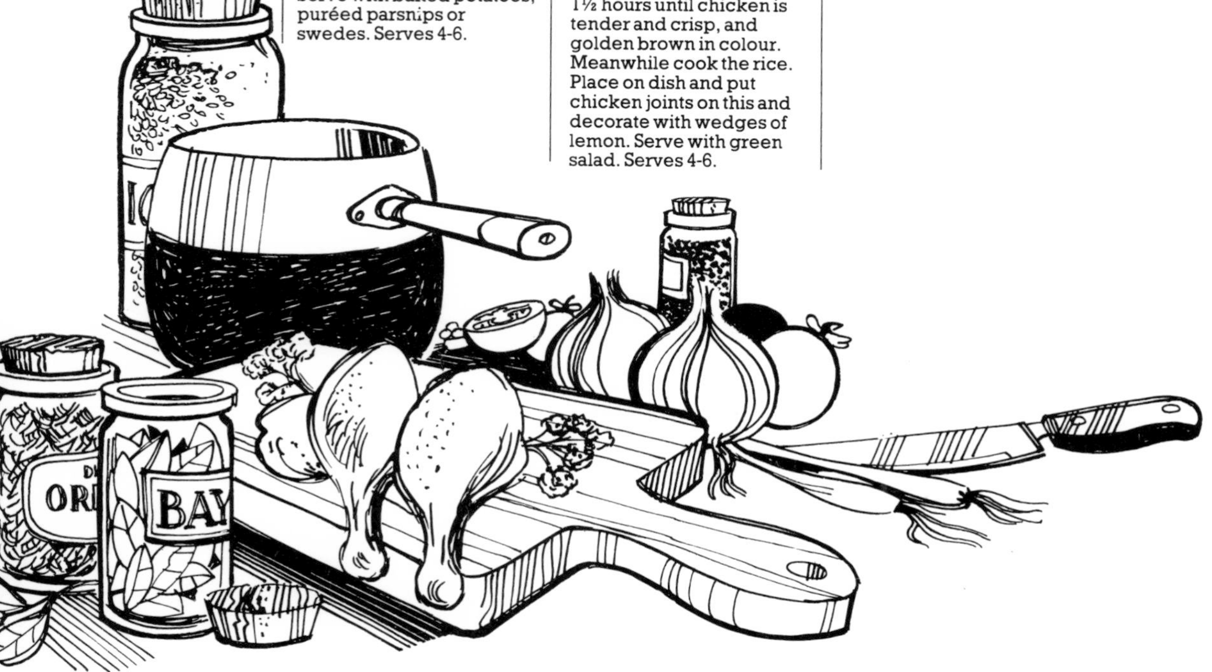

QUICK LIGHT MEALS

The second or light meal of the day should take the minimum time to prepare as it is usually taken at the busiest time. However the time saved in preparation should not be echoed by the time spent actually eating it. Food rushed is usually not appreciated and often it seems hardly to have existed! We need to make sure that every meal we take is an occasion even if eating alone. If you have a sandwich, make it an open one and eat it with a knife and fork. If you have soup from a thermos, eat it from a bowl and add the garnishes from a separate container. Lay the table, set out a tray, take your time. Not only will you feel more satisfied, it will appeal to your other senses of sight, smell and feel as well. You are also likely to eat far less food! Try even in a snack meal to mix several foods – breads, vegetables with egg, meat or cheese in some of the following ways:

Open Sandwiches The ideas for these are numerous and can be based on the salad ideas together with the many different cottage cheeses on the market these days. Pickles of many sorts can also be used. If the topping is moist you will not need butter or margarine.

Soups Again can be taken from our list or added to by ideas of your own. Watch the ones you buy from the shops and read your labels carefully to check for salt and sugar. Make a meal of it by serving with a wholemeal roll.

Yoghurt Can add up to many variations. Try Greta's favourite: Soak 1 tbsp each of rolled oats, dessicated coconut and raisins in orange juice for 2 hours. Then add it to a 5.29oz (150g) carton of yoghurt with 2 grated carrots. This can be varied by using apple juice or walnuts, etc.

Another one from Scandinavia is: To a 5.29oz (150g) carton of yoghurt add a chopped pickled herring and a chopped soused herring, season with horseradish to taste. Serve with a salad.

Cottage Cheese This blends with a variety of additions apart from those already on the market. Try the pink lumpfish (Danish caviar!) for grand occasions, or add the strips of crab meat to be found in the delicatessen. Beat in garlic, fresh herbs, lemon juice or virtually anything which is low in fat or not containing refined carbohydrates. Cottage cheese can add bulk when you are trying to reduce high-calorie foods. Add chopped vegetables and serve with a crispbread.

Nibbles There are many different packets of high-fibre foods, such as different combinations of fruits and nuts, seeds and wholewheat crisps. These can be very useful for packed lunches especially for those requiring high-energy content such as children and the more active adults. Many of the snacks sold in health food shops are high in calories. Do remember to *read* the packets and watch the salt and sugar contents.

Fresh Fruit is an easy snack that needs no preparation.

Eggs These are very useful and can be dressed up in many ways. They can be boiled and served with the black lumpfish (Danish caviar). They can be hardboiled and filled with cottage cheese/chives/mashed tomatoes/curry, etc. They can be set in aspic and made to look pretty; they can be poached and eaten with spinach and a little cheese or on brown toast; they can be scrambled with a little skimmed milk cooked slowly in a greased non-stick pan and flavoured with horseradish.

Hungarian Cheese

1lb (450g) cottage cheese
½ tsp paprika
1 tsp each caraway seeds, mustard powder, chopped capers, chopped chives or spring onions
2 tbsp plain yoghurt
1 tbsp beer
Garnish: radishes and onions

Work the cottage cheese with a wooden spoon through a sieve into a large bowl. Mix in enough paprika to colour the cheese a faint pink. Blend in the caraway seeds, mustard, capers and chives or spring onions. Add the yoghurt and beer and mix all the ingredients until thoroughly distributed. If you do not wish to eat the cheese at once it will keep in the refrigerator for several days. Serve with wholemeal bread. Serves 4-6.

Welsh Eggs

per person:
2 med cooked leeks (including green leaves)
2 mashed potatoes
1 egg
2 dstsp plain yoghurt
Pinch of Parmesan, freshly milled black pepper

Mash the leeks and potatoes with the pepper until they are a pale green colour. Put in a lightly-greased small oven-proof dish. Make a well and break the egg into it. Cover with the yoghurt and sprinkle with the Parmesan. Bake in a hot oven until the egg is set.

Instead of the leeks you can use:
Parsnip flavoured with orange juice
Cauliflower purée (cook in skimmed milk) flavoured with a pinch of nutmeg
Carrot and caraway seed purée
Brussel sprout and chestnut purée
All the above can be used as vegetables and sauces.

DESSERTS

It may seem strange that we include a section on desserts in a book dedicated to good health. However a dish designed to finish a meal with a sweet taste does not automatically fall into the 'bad for you' category. It is quite easy to create excellent and delicious recipes which use natural ingredients that are high in roughage, low in fat and without sugar. However, keep desserts for special occasions and certainly not more than once or twice a week as they are (albeit very pleasant) extra! It is important for those of you who need to lose or control your weight to realise that because of their very sweet nature (and fat in some cases) these recipes are naturally high in calories and should be avoided or at best limited until your weight has come down to target. Having a special meal once a week is good for the soul so perhaps you could try them on these occasions. These recipes are naturally only a few of those you can try. Look out for healthy eating books on the market (make sure they abide by the rules) and adapt other recipes. As a general rule, instead of these desserts, use fruits (especially some of the exotic ones) to finish a meal.

Strawberry Soufflé

3 lvl tsp powdered gelatine
4 tbsp orange juice
8oz (225g) clean, hulled strawberries
¼ pt (140ml) plain low-fat yoghurt
3 egg whites whipped until stiff but not dry

Put the gelatine and orange juice in the top of a double saucepan over hot water, or in cup standing in a pan of hot water. Set over low heat and stir the gelatine until it dissolves. Set the liquid aside to cool. Mash or liquidise the strawberries, stir in the gelatine mixture and fold in the yoghurt. Cover the bowl and put in a refrigerator for about 10 minutes so that the gelatine just begins to set. Fold in the whisked egg whites. Pile the soufflé high into a straight-sided souffle dish or into individual glasses. Put back in the refrigerator to set for 1 hour or more. Serves 4-6.

Spikey Pears

6 cooking pears or hard dessert pears
½ pt (285ml) sweet cider
Thinly-pared rind of half a small lemon
1oz (25g) blanched almonds, cut into slivers

Peel the pears thinly, but leave the stems on. Put into an oven-proof dish and cover with the cider. Add the lemon rind. Cover and cook in a pre-heated oven at Gas 2 (300°F/150°C) until tender. This may take 4 hours or longer. Leave the pears to cool in the liquid and then lift out carefully into shallow serving dish. Stand upright pressed together. Press the almond slivers all over the fruit. Reduce the liquid by boiling fast over a high heat. Pour over the fruit and serve with brown bread ice. Serves 6.

Bread and Fruit Pudding

2oz (50g) glacé cherries
4oz (100g) sultanas
2fl.oz (50ml) fresh orange juice or sherry
10 slices wholemeal bread
4 eggs
1 pt (570ml) skimmed milk

Set the oven to Gas 4 (350°F/180°C). Quarter the cherries and mix with the sultanas. Cover with orange juice or sherry. Cut each slice of bread into triangles. Arrange half the triangles in a shallow oven-proof dish which has been lightly greased. Sprinkle with half the dried fruit and arrange the remaining triangles on top. Sprinkle the rest of the dried fruit over. Beat the eggs and skimmed milk together and pour over the bread. Bake for 40-45 minutes. Serves 6.

Pink Grapefruit and Mint Sorbet

2 large grapefruit (if possible the pink variety) peeled, de-pipped, devoid of pith and blended
1 tsp muscovado sugar
¼ pt (140ml) water
3 sprigs mint
1 egg white

Boil the sugar and water until the sugar has dissolved. Put the mint into the syrup and leave off the heat for 20 minutes. Strain and leave to cool. Mix with the grapefruit pulp and put into a rigid container and freeze until semi-frozen, about 45 minutes to 1 hour. Beat the egg white in a bowl until it is stiff. Fold it into the sorbet and return it to the freezer until frozen to a firm mush, about 1 hour. Serve in glasses and decorate with mint leaves.

Brown Bread Ice

4 large slices of wholemeal bread
3oz (75g) muscovado sugar
15.9oz (450g) carton low-fat plain yoghurt

Reduce the bread to fine breadcrumbs and mix with brown sugar. Spread the crumbs on a lightly oiled baking tray and put this into the centre of an oven, preheated to Gas 6 (400°F/200°C). Leave until the sugar caramelises and the crumbs are golden brown; stir them occasionally. Leave to cool, then break up into crumbs again with a fork. Drain the yoghurt of any excess liquid. Stir in the breadcrumb mixture and put into shallow freezing tray. Cover and put in freezer until it is firm.

Baked Stuffed Apples

6 large cooking apples, cored
4fl.oz (125ml) sherry
Fillings:
2 large bananas, peeled and mashed with lemon juice
or 6oz (175g) dried apricots, chopped and mixed with honey
or 6oz (175g) mincemeat (make your own without suet)
or 3oz (175g) dried dates, chopped with 3oz (75g) mixed nuts and juice of a lemon

Score the skin round each apple and stand them in a deep, lightly-oiled oven-proof dish. Fill the cavities with the chosen filling, pour the sherry round the fruit and bake in a pre-heated oven Gas 4 (350°F/180°C) for 1 hour. Baste occasionally. Serve hot or cold.

Carrot Cake

4oz (100g) wholemeal flour
2 tsp baking powder
2fl.oz (50ml) corn oil
2oz (50g) muscovado sugar
1 tsp cinnamon
½ tsp vanilla essence
7oz (200g) carrots grated
2 eggs beaten
2oz (50g) walnuts chopped

Preset the oven to Gas 4 (350°F/180°C). Put 1oz grated carrot to one side. Mix all the other ingredients together. Put into an oiled and lined 8-inch (20-cm) diameter cake tin. Bake for 45 minutes to 1 hour, or until firm to the touch. Sprinkle with grated carrot. Serves 6.

Fruit Salad

2 oranges peeled and chopped into large pieces
2 red-skinned apples thinly sliced
2 bananas sliced
4 of the following: 1 chopped pear, 1 small punnet strawberries (hulled and halved if large), 4oz (100g) black or green grapes (halved and deseeded), or 2oz (50g) sultanas, 1 peach sliced
Orange juice

Mix all ingredients together and cover with fresh orange juice. Serve with low-fat, plain yoghurt. Serves 6.

Blackberry Sorbet

1½ pts (850ml) water
1lb (450g) blackberries
Juice of one lemon or orange if you like it sweeter
Whites of 2 eggs

Slowly cook the blackberries in the water until the juice runs. Turn off the heat and leave for 30 minutes. Sieve and remove the pips, stir in the lemon juice. Turn into a container and cool. Freeze for 1 hour until semi-frozen. Beat the egg whites in a bowl until firm though not stiff. Fold into the sorbet and freeze again until firm (about 1 hour). Serve in wine glasses and decorate with a mint leaf.

LOW-CALORIE MENU A

Approx. 1,000 calories

Daily allowance: ½ pint (284ml) skimmed milk

	BREAKFAST (approx 200 cals)	LIGHT MEAL (approx 400 cals)	MAIN MEAL (approx 400 cals)
MON	Unsweetened high-fibre breakfast cereal. Skimmed milk (from allowance). Glass fruit juice.	4oz tub cottage cheese (seasoned), mixed with chopped raw veg (e.g. carrot, onion, pepper. 4 Ryvita. Piece of fruit (e.g. banana).	Chicken Veronique*. Brown rice salad (tomato and cucumber).
TUES	Half grapefruit. Poached or boiled egg. Slice wholemeal toast with low-fat spread, Marmite or Bovril.	Low-calorie vegetable soup (e.g. Leek soup). Slice wholemeal toast with low-calorie spread. Slice of melon.	Spanish omelette*. Poached mushrooms. 2 crispbreads. Fresh fruit (e.g. orange).
WED	Natural yoghurt with diced fresh fruit (according to season). Slice wholemeal toast with low-fat spread.	Wholemeal herb scones (2). Low-fat spread plus salad vegetables as filling or accompaniment (lettuce, tomato, cucumber, etc). Piece of fruit.	Savoury-mince-stuffed vegetable (Marrow, onion or pepper)*. 1 tablespoonful frozen peas. Baked apple (sweetened with teaspoon honey and cinnamon).
THURS	Grapefruit and orange (Florida cocktail). High-fibre breakfast cereal and skimmed milk from allowance.	Small can of tuna mixed with seasoned natural yoghurt, tomato and cucumber. Wholemeal roll or bread. Piece of fruit (e.g. apple).	Browned tomatoes. Cabbage (lightly cooked and flavoured with black pepper and/or dill). Low-fat fruit yoghurt.
FRI	Bran cereal with fresh fruit (or prunes) and milk from allowance. Glass fruit juice.	1 chopped hard-boiled egg mixed with low-calorie mayonnaise (flavour with curry powder or tomato paste). 4 wholewheat crispbreads. Piece of fruit.	Spaghetti with lentils. Lemon surprise*.
SAT	½ grapefruit. Slice wholemeal toast with low-fat spread.	Large baked potato with cottage cheese and chives (or low-calorie choice filling). Piece of fruit (e.g. Tangerine).	Kedgeree*. Grilled tomatoes. Fresh fruit salad.
SUN	Fruit juice. Poached or boiled egg. Slice wholemeal toast with low-fat spread.	Cottage cheese open sandwiches. (Cottage cheese plus celery, tomato, cucumber, pineapple, etc). Fruit (e.g. banana).	Grilled lamb chop with tomato. Potatoes mashed with skimmed milk. Mixed diced carrot and parsnip or broad beans. Fruit sorbet.

* Meals marked with an asterisk indicate their recipes follow

LOW-CALORIE MENU B

Approx. 1,200 calories

Daily allowance: ½ pint (284ml) skimmed milk

	BREAKFAST (approx 200 cals)	**LIGHT MEAL (approx 400 cals)**	**MAIN MEAL (approx 400-600 cals)**
MON	High-fibre breakfast cereal with skimmed milk or natural yoghurt *or* Slice wholemeal bread with low-fat spread, Marmite or Bovril.	Low-calorie vegetable soup. Mushroom or onion (vegetables simmered in stock – no fat). Slice wholemeal toast with low-calorie spread. Fruit (e.g. banana).	Fish bake*. Jacket potato, baked tomatoes. Spiced pears*.
TUES	Fruit juice. *or* Portion of canned fruit without added sugar. *or* Portion fresh fruit.	Blue cheese dip*. Half piece of pitta bread. Fruit (e.g. apple).	Greek spiced ring with 'Slimmers' Kebabs*. Portion of fresh fruit.
WED	High-fibre breakfast cereal with skimmed milk or natural yoghurt. *or* Slice wholemeal bread with low-fat spread.	Egg and cress savoury (hardboiled egg, mustard and cress, seasoned yoghurt dressing). 4 wholewheat crispbreads. Fruit (e.g. orange).	Haricot or kidney beans baked with tomatoes, onion and 1oz Edam cheese. 4oz (100g) baked potato. Fruit (e.g. apple).
THURS	Fruit juice. *or* Portion of canned fruit without added sugar. *or* Portion of fresh fruit.	Slice of melon. 2 cold roast chicken drumsticks. Mixed salad with vinaigrette dressing (olive oil, lemon juice, garlic, mustard, thyme and sage – blended).	Spinach soufflé. Seasonal salad vegetables. Slice wholemeal bread and low-calorie spread. Fruit salad with yoghurt.
FRI	High-fibre breakfast cereal with skimmed milk or natural yoghurt.	Cottage cheese salad (seasonal salad vegetables). Wholemeal rolls or bread. Fresh fruit.	Leeks in blankets*. Grilled tomatoes. Fresh fruit.
SAT	Boiled or poached egg. *or* Grilled kipper. *or* Single rasher lean grilled bacon, if desired.	Small can baked beans (add extra flavour with curry powder, extra tomato, etc). Slice wholemeal toast (low-calorie spread). Fruit (e.g. apple).	Fisherman's chowder. Low calorie jelly*.
SUN	Slice wholemeal bread with low-fat spread, Marmite or Bovril. Glass fruit juice.	Low-calorie soup (own choice). 4 wholewheat crispbreads, with low-calorie spread. Piece of fruit (e.g. banana).	Roast chicken, thin gravy (e.g. oxo). Green beans, carrots, boiled potatoes. Melon and ginger whip*.

* Meals marked with an asterisk indicate their recipes follow

Low-Calorie Recipes

*Leeks in Blankets
(or cauliflower/asparagus etc)

8 med leeks (cauliflower or asparagus)
8 slices cooked ham (lean and thinly sliced)
2 tbsp dried skimmed milk or fresh
2 tsp cornflour
Seasoning
Parsley or Parmesan cheese

Use 2 pieces of ham and 2 leeks per person. Boil vegetable until just tender in minimum water. Strain and reserve stock. Mix stock with skimmed milk and thicken slightly with cornflour. Season well. Place thin slices of ham over vegetables (or wrap around leeks) in an ovenproof dish. Pour over the sauce and top with fine sprinkling of Parmesan cheese. (Alternatively, make parsley sauce by adding chopped parsley). Serves 4.

*Melon and Ginger Whip

1 small melon
1 orange
2 egg whites
½ oz (17g) gelatine
Powdered ginger to taste

Grate zest of orange and squeeze the juice. Dissolve gelatine in the orange juice. Allow to cool then liquidise with the melon flesh and orange zest to give a smooth pulp. Refrigerate until on the point of setting, fold in the stiffly whisked egg whites. Spoon into individual dishes and sprinkle on powdered ginger before serving. Serves 4.

*Low-Calorie Jelly

3 tsp gelatine
9fl.oz (250ml) orange juice (unsweetened)
1 orange
4oz (100g) halved strawberries

Put the gelatine in the orange juice and heat until dissolved. When cooled down add the fruit and leave to set. Any combinations of fruit may be used. Serves 4.

*Chicken Veronique

2oz (50g) cooked chicken
2oz (50g) black or green grapes
Juice and rind of 1 lemon
2 tbsp yoghurt (natural)
Watercress to garnish

Mix diced chicken and halved grapes. In a separate container mix lemon rind and juice with yoghurt and season to taste. Pour over chicken and grapes and toss well. Serves 1.

*Spanish Omelette

1 small onion thinly sliced
2 medium eggs
1 chopped tomato
1 small green pepper, finely sliced
Pinch dried thyme, black pepper
Fresh parsley to garnish

Lightly grease pan with olive oil and cook onion. Add other vegetables and cook for 5 minutes, stirring often. Stir in seasonings. Whisk eggs and pour over vegetables in the pan. Cook slowly until egg is set and put under grill to brown the top. Serves 1.

*Savoury Mince Stuffing

2oz (50g) lean minced beef
7oz (200g) canned tomatoes
2oz (50g) thinly sliced vegetables (e.g. carrot, celery)
½ beef stock cube
1 tbsp cooked rice

Cook mince in a non-stick pan, stirring over a low heat. When browned, add vegetables and stir until cooked. Add tomatoes and beef stock cube. Add seasoning and herbs to taste. Mix with cooked rice. Stuff pepper (marrow or onion) and bake at Gas 6 (400°F/200°C) for 30 minutes. Serves 1.

*Kedgeree

2oz (50g) cooked brown rice
1 small onion
1 tbsp sweetcorn
6oz (150g) cooked kippers
1 tbsp skimmed milk
1 hard boiled egg
2 tbsp chopped parsley
Freshly ground black pepper
Knob of vegetable margarine

Peel and finely chop onion. Stir fry gently till soft with margarine. Add rice, flaked cooked fish, chopped egg and sweetcorn. Add seasoning to taste. Finally stir in the milk and chopped parsley, reserving a little for garnish. Serves 1.

*Fish Bake

1lb (450g) cod
4oz (125g) mushrooms
1 large onion
Lemon

Season fish with salt and pepper. Place on kitchen foil. Thinly slice onions and mushrooms and place on top of fish. Add a squeeze of lemon. Seal foil and bake at Gas 4 (350°F/ 180°C) for 30-40 minutes. Serve garnished with lemon. Serves 4.

N.B. Try serving baked fish with baked banana sprinkled with lemon juice.

*Spiced Pears (or Apples)

1 large orange
1 lemon
1lb (450g) dessert pears (apples)
¼ tsp ground ginger

Squeeze juice from orange and lemon. Sieve. Put in saucepan with 2 tablespoons water and ginger. Peel and core pears (apples). Cut in half and add to pan. Bring to boil. Cover and simmer for 20 minutes. Pour liquid over pears in serving dish and chill. Serves 4.

*Blue Cheese Dip

2oz (50g) Danish blue cheese
2oz (50g) natural yoghurt
Seasoning

Blend all ingredients and chill. Use sliced raw vegetables to dip, e.g. carrot, cabbage, celery, peppers, cauliflower. Serves 4-6.

*Slimmers Kebabs

Quantity depends on numbers.
Small cubes liver or kidney
Small cubes lean beef, lamb, pork, veal or chicken
Small peeled onions
Halved tomatoes
Button mushrooms
Small pieces of lean rolled bacon
Green or red peppers
Cubes fresh pineapple
Seasonings of curry or ginger powder
Salt and pepper
Oil, sunflower
(Weigh the meat used for the kebabs and count the calories)

Thread each skewer with alternate pieces of meat and vegetables or fruit. Mix seasonings with small quantity of sunflower oil to brush meat and vegetables. Cook under a hot grill, turning frequently for 10-15 minutes or until cooked.

*Lemon Surprise

2 lemons rind and juice
2-3 eggs
½ oz (17g) gelatine
Liquid sweetener

Place lemon rind in half pint of water and bring to boil. Strain lemon rind and water into lemon juice. Place gelatine in three tablespoons cold water in a basin. Place basin over saucepan of water over moderate heat and stir until gelatine dissolves. Add gelatine and sweetener to water and lemon rind. Stir until dissolved and leave in cool place until almost set. Add egg whites and whisk until mixture has doubled in volume. Pour into individual glasses and leave to set. Serves 4.

SECTION 3

RELAXATION

Tension Control is easy to understand, easy to put into practice and achieves the desired results. The technique works on the premise that only a fully contracted muscle will fully relax when it is released and that whereas tight muscles signal to the brain that there is an 'alert' to be responded to, relaxed muscles have the opposite effect. It does not need special apparatus, a dark quiet place or another person or teacher, to put it into operation. You can use it at any time, in any situation and in particular when you feel that tension is getting out of control.

Learning Tension Control is an essential aid to living well, for however many ways you can manage to learn to relax, it is also important to have a skill on which you can call on during 'stress moments' or in times of crisis. Over the years the members of our Slimnastics classes and many others have found the Neuromuscular Technique or Tension Control to be the vital clue to easier, less troubled and more effective living.

During the six-week programme you will become familiar with the Tension Control Technique, and once you have learned it you will be able to put it into operation when you need it. To become familiar with the Tension Control Technique, you need to:

- Read and memorise and feel the technique
- Then look and watch yourself in practice.
- Next think and recognise any tension in yourself.
- Feel the results as you put the technique into operation.
- Listen to your own rhythm and try the sleep exercises.
- Practise continually until it becomes almost automatic.

To understand how and why this form of relaxation works it will help to look at the reactions and effects of stress and tension on the body.

RELAXATION

Tension and the Body

The 'Red Alert' Response

Watch a rabbit in a field when it senses a 'presence' – it sits up, the ears stretch high, the nose twitches and the eyes are bright as frozen for a moment, it assesses the situation. If it's another male impinging on already marked territory, the rabbit springs forward to thump the ground and see off the enemy; if it's a human, the rabbit shows its white bobtail and back feet as a warning to the others before disappearing down the burrow. Occasionally, it's a false alarm, but to make sure the rabbit drops down and becomes motionless until once more it can relax and carry on eating. Think of your response when walking home through a dark street and you suddenly become aware that someone might be following you; your expression freezes, your ears almost feel they are stretching backwards as you locate the sounds 'how near are they? are they menacing?', you might feel angry and turn to face the oncomer or more likely run away out of the suspected danger; just occasionally you might feel 'rooted to the spot' until you feel secure again. These responses are the natural and very necessary defences we need for self preservation.

Your whole body is affected by this 'red alert' response; the sense organs, most frequently those of sight or hearing, receive the signal of alarm and pass it on to the brain where its significance is recognised and from which messages are sent along the nerves to the muscles and to other organs. The muscles contract, often very abruptly as in the startled response. If the state of alertness or arousal continues, muscle activity and tension remain high and enable you to be more capable of reacting quickly to any further alert.

The signal from the eyes and ears to the brain and on to the muscles which in turn contract into tension, triggers:

A changed heart rate which is usually increased (most people know the feeling of the fast beating heart after a near miss when driving!). However some people in anticipation of shock or unpleasantness feel their heart beat slowing down and beating forcibly.

A rise in blood pressure often to a very high level that can remain so for some time.

An effect on the blood vessels throughout the body: those in the muscle open up so that more blood can course through them; those in the abdomen and in the skin contract; so that less blood goes through them. The output of the heart is diverted from the skin and gut to the muscle of the trunk and limbs in preparation for greater muscular effort. As a direct cause of this, you become very pale and the stomach becomes flabby, giving you a heavy 'sinking' feeling.

An increase in sweating in fairly specific areas such as the skin around the mouth and nose, the temples, the arm-pits, between the legs and especially the palms of the hands and the soles of the feet. The nervous public speaker can literally stream with perspiration.

A drying up of the saliva and an increase in the secretion of gastric acid; the gastro-intestinal tract is markedly affected although movements of the stomach may diminish. The intestines are more active and may churn and gurgle. You may feel an urge to open your bowels. The bladder is similarly affected and there is an urge to pass water as the bladder muscle increases in its activity. We all recognise the constant need to visit the toilet before an interview or important meeting.

The dilation of the pupil of your eye which lets in more light and helps it to function in a more sensitive manner. Your other senses are similarly affected.

An expansion of the breathing tubes (bronchi) which allows more air to be drawn into the lungs.

A change in your hormones. These are less immediate because their speed is determined by the rate of the blood's circulation round the body. Hormones are chemical substances which are secreted into the blood stream by glands in various places throughout the body and travel in the blood stream to their particular sites of action. Many hormones are implicated in stress responses, the most important ones are adrenaline and noradrenaline, and cortisol or hydrocortisone (an adrenocortical hormone). Different species of animals secrete adrenaline and noradrenaline in different proportions. In man it is mainly adrenaline and when this and noradrenaline are secreted into the bloodstream they act on many organs and reinforce all the above effects. In addition, adrenaline influences the metabolic balance of the body, mobilising energy reserves in the liver and in the muscles themselves, making glucose available for immediate energy demands.

You are now ready for ACTION!

The 'Constant' Tension Response

But what happens if you are unable to respond with any 'action' when your body is fully prepared and ready? – there you are lying beneath the bed clothes convinced there is a burglar downstairs, your heart beats, your blood pressure rises, you grow pale, your pupils dilate, you breathe faster, feel butterflies in your stomach and your mouth is dry; you start to tremble and want to go to the 'loo', but you dare not move. Similarly day after day the boss or committee might thwart some plans which you have painstakingly worked out and considered and because of your less advanced position you have to accept their decision, clench your fists, grit your teeth and go back to the drawing board again! Likewise, quarrelling, anxiety, decisions, deadlines and of course many more occasions and feelings leave you with your responses 'pent up' and with no outlet. Your tension reactions have most likely set in motion all the 'red alert' responses, but because the appropriate response in each case *isn't* to run and burn off the reaction, you are left instead with all the added chemicals flooding your body.

Everyone has an individual pattern of physiological and psychological response to an 'alert' and this pattern will tend to be repeated when another signal comes. This means that one person may show a marked increase in heart beat each time while sweating only very little, another may perspire profusely; one person might show a rise in blood pressure, another an increase in gastric acid, or perhaps severe muscle tension. We develop, and increasingly develop, our own particular physical reactions to these calls on our energies.

This results in our developing our own physical warning signals when tension has reached an uncontrollable level; you might recognise one or some of these physiological symptoms:

- Throbbing head or headache.
- Grinding teeth, impacted nerve.
- Twitching eyes, tremulous voice.
- Pain spreading up the neck over the back of the head.
- Tightness in the throat, a feeling of choking.
- Overbreathing (hyperventilation).
- Aches between the shoulder blades.
- Nail biting, damaged cuticles, twiddling thumbs.
- Palpitations and chest discomfort.
- Skin rashes.
- Vomiting and indigestion.

- Diarrhoea and frequency of urination.
- Backache in general, especially in the lower back.
- Tiredness, weakness, sweating, trembling, breathlessness, fainting or insomnia.

Our psychological symptoms can include:

- Increase in smoking.
- Increase in alcohol intake.
- A marked increase or decrease in appetite.
- Inability, or constant desire and ability to sleep.
- Feelings of tiredness and exhaustion.
- Absent-mindedness, inefficiency, loss of interest, lack of concentration.
- Loss of sex drive.
- Feelings of inability to cope.
- Irritability, impulsiveness, loss of co-ordination.
- Depression

All these can be a reaction to stress. Of course some of them may be the symptoms of another cause but if you have checked that you are not ill and you frequently experience one of these reactions you should take heed. They are your warning signals as to when excess tension is making your body suffer. They may be unpleasant but they are useful.

Stress-Related Diseases

Your 'locked in' response to tension and the corresponding physical reactions can contribute to actual bodily illness. Some illnesses are believed to be directly related, at least in part, to tension. In some forms of tension, reaction to stress seems to be the most important factor. In others this 'over' stress is not the major factor but can make the condition worse or make bouts of illness more likely. Some stress-related diseases are:

Allergies An allergy is an abnormally sensitive reaction to a substance which is in itself normally not harmful: these reactions may be hay fever, itching, rashes, streaming eyes, joint pains, wheezing. Some but not all, sufferers find that their attacks are more frequent or more severe under conditions of stress; in some cases, emotion may be the principal factor.

Alopecia is baldness in which the hair falls out in handfuls and this includes not only scalp hair but eyebrows and body hair as well. The cause is uncertain but some sufferers can relate it to episodes of stress. It also occurs as a result of hormone imbalance such as that caused by childbirth.

Asthma is not caused by stress but in some people it is the initiating factor; in others stress is the factor which prolongs the attack. Often it is a combination of factors that produces an attack. Also the worse the breathlessness, the greater is the feeling of anxiety which in turn may prolong or worsen the attack.

Cancer In spite of a great deal of research much remains to be discovered about the causes of cancer. It is most likely that like heart attacks there is no single cause rather a combination of risk factors. There is a theory that emotional factors could be a contributing factor in some cancers. Cancer is beginning to be seen as one of the diseases in which the functioning of the body may become affected by physical changes associated with upset mental and emotional processes. It has for instance been strongly indicated that people who suppress their emotions, such as anger and hostility, are more likely to be cancer prone.

Diabetes is unlikely to be caused by either physical or emotional stress. It is however thought to be sometimes triggered off by physical illness, injury or emotional upset and can affect the severity for the sufferer.

Migraine is a specific type of headache caused by spasms and relaxations of the blood vessels in the coverings of the brain. Again there are many causes but some sufferers recognise that their attacks are closely related to periods of stress and tension in their lives.

Pain is very subjective; no one can truly feel the pain of anyone else. However it is certain that already existing pain can become worse under stress and tension, for by its very nature of prolonged contraction of muscles leading in some cases to severe spasm, it can cause very real physical pain (such as the neck ache experienced by so many after a stressful drive).

Peptic Ulcers have several different causes but acid appears to play a leading role. The stomach usually produces a strong acid but protects itself from being digested by this acid by secreting a coating of mucus. Stress increases the secretion of acid and decreases the secretion of mucus. Although ulcers can be healed by medicine they can often return if the sufferer does not modify his life style and alleviate the stress as well as changing his diet, avoiding spirits and giving up smoking.

Rheumatoid Arthritis has been linked with stress either with its onset or by a worsening when it occurs. It has been found that in the three months before onset of the disease many sufferers have been through significantly stressful life events. The specific cause of the inflammatory reaction is not clear. It seems likely that as in the case of cancer, the body's immune mechanisms, which normally play an important part in the defence of the body against disease, are disturbed so that they are activated by some of the body's own protein producing destruction and inflammation.

Skin Diseases are not primarily of emotional origin, however stress and tension play an important part in the development, aggravation and perpetuation of many of them such as urticaria, itching in the anogenital region, acne, atopic eczema and psoriasis. Also the stress and misery caused by the skin disease may create a vicious circle.

It is not difficult to see that there is a great deal to be gained in learning to cope with stress and the control of your tension. This can be achieved in many ways and some of them need the help of others to be really effective. Do not hesitate to seek professional help from doctors, counsellors, or other trained guidance bodies should you feel the need. We have concentrated here on the steps you can take for yourself. They are simple and straightforward and they work! However relaxation is a *skill* and as such it has to be practised and learned and success does not come overnight! Remember though – it is in your interest to learn tension control; it is a skill none of us can afford to be without so now is the time to start.

ACHIEVING RELAXATION

Achieving Relaxation
Everyone can benefit from learning relaxation techniques: athletes need it to perfect their abilities, thinkers to increase their concentration, performers to release their energies and sensitive people to aid their protection. Even normally relaxed people with seemingly not a care in the world can benefit and should not neglect to practise this skill. In the first place they may well need to use it in times of emergencies and without the skill they will have nothing to fall back on, and in the second they should examine what they think of as truly relaxed. The human body can never be truly relaxed unless it is lying flat! It needs some tension just to keep upright: the muscle tone keeps the spine supported and posture alert and lively; some tension is necessary to stimulate your hormones and keep you alive, thinking and awake. This tension may be only slight, spontaneous and undemanding but if you remember the section about muscles it is obvious that a muscle has to be first fully contracted before it can completely relax. It is therefore arguable that people who never experience real tension never fully release it! It may be that 'laid back' people need tension control more than they think.

It is the same with people who have learned to ignore or be unaware of stress factors to the extent that they no longer respond physically to them: for instance people living under a flight path often cease to notice the noise of the aircraft, or those living near a busy road or near a factory who do not notice the noise of traffic or machinery. Adaptation like this is a complex matter and its mechanism in warding off the effects of stress is not fully known, but it is possible that the tension is just registered by the person but not responded to, resulting in complex nervous system changes such as those in the sensitivity of the hormonal control mechanisms. These people too need to master these true relaxation techniques.

There are several steps everyone can take to help themselves.

Exercise!
If it is the fully stretched muscle which can completely relax then any exercise that involves the whole body in 'mobilising', 'pulsing-up' and 'toning-up' will do the trick. The Slimnastics Exercise Programme which incorporates all these stages is therefore in itself positive relaxation. But there are other ways too . . . **walk more often** for a start! Not idling though, it must be brisk! Walk everywhere you can; leave the car at home, forget the bus or at least go on to the next stop and enjoy some fresh air. When you walk make sure your posture is good. In particular make sure that your head is well balanced and your neck stretched as part of the spine; keep the eyes looking forward. Then place the first foot gently on the ground in front and push onto it using the ball of the foot behind (this involves considerable ankle work from the second leg); swing the arms gently. Practise this way of walking, it lessens the strain, quickens the pace automatically and looks graceful and gliding.

Swimming is one of the very best sports to achieve not only a fully exercised but also a relaxed body. However to do most good it is important to swim well and regularly. To this end more and more adults are attending swimming classes and gaining a great deal of pleasure at the same time. Swimming has the highest rating of all activities in improving suppleness, stamina and strength, it also stretches the body as well as supporting it so that there is no undue strain on any limbs or joints.

Other sports which can help are badminton, squash, basket ball, jogging or running but it is essential to mobilise and warm the body first. Too many tense people rush straight into exercise and this does far more harm than good.

Diverting your 'Mind'
If we concentrate on something which interests us or gives us pleasure, sometimes our brain will send messages to the muscles that all is well and that they can relax their anticipation. You have to force yourself to stop 'hanging on' to your tension which you might be doing in order to 'pay back' those who are guilty of causing you the strain! Maintaining long periods of silence after an argument or harbouring feelings of resentment affects other people far less than it affects yourself. Take some positive steps and enjoy feeling better; take responsibility for yourself and your happiness instead of being passive and waiting for others to do it for you – and being disappointed.

Music can be a superb soother and tranquilliser, it can also release inhibitions and raise the spirits – it is even better if you move because movement is almost a necessity for draining off the chemicals aroused by the tension, so dancing and singing can be very therapeutic. Playing an instrument too is excellent and conductors have a job which holds the claim for the highest lifespan (if you watch a conductor at work you will see how active, agile, and totally involved he is as well as being probably of advanced years!).

Learning something new, reading, writing all can be helpful. So can a change of environment, holidays, visits, being at home or going out to work, all these may help the 'soul'. Having a bath in warm water is comforting and having a shower is stimulating and refreshing.

Talking to a friend, neighbour or member of the family can help you see your problems in perspective. If you really feel unable to cope yourself, talking to a skilled counsellor may be very helpful.

Massage is one of the most ancient forms of natural healing. You massage yourself naturally then you rub any part of the body you have hurt. Massage can ease away tension and even gently unknot a tense muscle which has gone into spasm. A really good body massage is both a pleasurable and therapeutic experience and probably best when given by a professional. However there are basic movements you can do yourself particularly on the most vulnerable and helpful spots such as the neck and feet.

Your body should be warm and comfortable before you start (after your bath would be ideal); use a body oil on your hands to keep your movements smooth and avoid any inflamed area. If you are massaging your neck and shoulders, place your hands on either side of the neck palms downwards, and gently knead the muscles on either side of the spine working down to the nape. (*always work towards the heart* when massaging any area), repeat this until you feel relaxed. Now glide your finger tips hand over hand down from the nape of the neck to the shoulders and repeat this action, kneading any 'knots' of muscle spasm if necessary. For your feet work towards the heart by finger kneading from toes to ankle. Knead your soles as well but this time with the heel of your palm (according to the science of Reflexology this helps other parts of the body as well). Now stroke your fingertips, hand after hand, up the leg from ankle to knee. By the time you have finished all these actions you will be warm, relaxed and exercised!

Meditation using a form of chant to focus the mind until a trance-like state is achieved lowers the blood pressure dramatically. There are several different techniques and they do need to be taught and mastered. Meditation needs to be practised in a warm atmosphere for at least ten to fifteen minutes in quiet and solitude. There should be total concentration with no thought of ordinary existence.

There is another form of meditation which can be mastered on your own and which can give you a more positive outcome. Again you do need to be quiet and peaceful and able to lie down in comfort and safety. Close your eyes and gently place your palms on your stomach (below the waist), breathe in until you feel your hands rise and continue until you can take in no more air, hold the position and then allow the air to come rushing out, hold for a moment and then repeat. When you feel really relaxed, your mind will find itself free and maybe even a trifle bored! Now, rehearse in your mind a skill you want to practise; go through the imagined movements carefully one by one until completed. You may be surprised the effect they have on your performance. The American tennis players use this method to great advantage.

Sleep is essential to your well-being. Without it you can become tense and nervous and when you are anxious and stressed you can suffer from insomnia. It can become a vicious circle. Sleep not only refreshes the body it also, through dreams, restores the mind and discharges tension.

The body works on a 24-hour cycle (everyone has their own inner clock known as a circadian rhythm), a cycle in which a 90- to 120-minute period of sleep – or wakefulness – alternates with a 5- to 10-minute dream period. It goes on unceasingly 24 hours a day and it is combined with a similar rise and fall of the body's temperature. The highest points are when you feel most alive and alert and the lowest when you are day-dreaming or sleep-dreaming. It is much easier to get to sleep during one of the low points in temperature; it is worth trying to keep track of them and adjust your sleep pattern accordingly if this is possible.

When you fall asleep, the eyelids close and the pupils become small. Breathing is diminished, blood pressure falls, the heart slows down, the temperature drops and the digestive juices and saliva decrease. There are several stages from drowsiness to oblivious sleep where all the muscles are relaxed and it is difficult to be woken. The brain still receives every sound and touch but though it responds, it does not express messages in actions (except in sleep walking). A normal person changes position from 20 to 60 times a night.

There are two kinds of sleep – slow wave sleep (which is dreamless and usually starts the sleeping sequence) and dreaming sleep, known as REM (Rapid Eye Movement). The two types alternate throughout the night. You will suffer little if you should be deprived of the slow-wave sleep but without REM you are likely to suffer increased tension and nervous reaction. REM sleep is the deepest and most refreshing; it is good for your mental health as it restores the central nervous system, though as to how this is achieved is not yet clear. Alcohol, barbiturates or tranquillizers all decrease the amount of REM sleep and may result in you waking up feeling depressed and tired.

So if you are longing for a good night's sleep yet you find yourself tossing and turning, and wide awake though tired, what steps can you take to help yourself clear your 'racing mind'? You might be busy reliving the minutiae of the day past, apprehensively surveying the day to come, or perhaps just worrying over details of almost no significance at all. First of all you must understand that your mental activity may well have triggered off a 'red alert' response. In that case it will be beneficial for you to get up and move – to the bathroom or to the kitchen – and then when you have cooled and calmed down, go back to bed and make yourself comfortable. Then quite deliberately:

- *Visualise* a room or a place where you feel safe and at home.
- *Look around* slowly and see the objects and the features (or people) if you have placed them there.
- *Look around again* faster this time.
- Repeat for a third time.
- Choose one point (an object, person or point) and keep your eyes fixed and try to think your way around.
- Do not let your eyes move (go back to the beginning if they do) but now repeat the thinking around again.
- You will fall asleep (if you do not cheat)!

This works because most people use their eye muscles and movements to 'visualise' their thoughts (you also verbalise thoughts or more often use a combination). However the majority cease to think when their eyes become fixed. An easy illustration of this is the number of people who fall fast asleep in front of television especially when the eyeline is static and even more so when the viewer is concentrating hard and really wants to hear and know what is being said! A lecturer can have the same effect.

A few more ideas Animals can help: dogs are companions, stroking a cat's fur can bring down the blood pressure. Gardening can be most satisfying – fulfilling our natural urge to till, grow and look after. Sex too can play its part. As a doctor in Hong Kong told the colony's Financial Women's Association 'sex is a good antidote to stress and tension' but he added 'the only problem is its inaccessibility in certain situations such as a traffic jam!' The Slimnastics Technique might prove more useful.

TENSION CONTROL TECHNIQUE

It sounds difficult memorising a 'technique' but in fact as you gradually become familiar with the moves and routine of our TCT (Tension Control Technique) the body will begin to automatically respond and eventually you will find yourself putting the technique into operation when needed, without conscious thought. However this eventual result does not just happen. It does need some concentration, time and thought to master this skill. For a skill it is; relaxation is not for most of us a natural habit, and so it has to be learned. But it is worth the practise and effort. To make it easy we will take it step by step:

- The first week we will ask you to concentrate on reading and 'doing' the technique.
- During the second week: reading, looking and 'doing'.
- You will then progress to thinking and recognising tension and release.
- By then you should be able to remember and feel the tension release.
- Next you will practise continually, and consciously apply the tension release during 'stress moments'.
- TCT should then become almost automatic.
- During the second six weeks you can also try the sleep exercises, deep meditation/relaxation, and massage as well.

The Tension Control Technique we use works on the premise that only a fully contracted muscle will fully relax when it is released; also that whereas tight muscles signal to the brain that there is an 'alert' to be responded to, relaxed muscles have the opposite effect. It is a simple straightforward idea, the beauty of it is that it works! To fully release any tension you have in your body you work steadily from the top to the toes, clenching the groups of muscles tightly, holding them and then releasing completely. Give yourself time to really feel the tension and then savour the relaxation with each move.

Before you start you will need to make sure you are in a position to be able to relax without any effort (for instance to stay upright or even in the chair). You should be able to breathe easily (no constricting clothes or slumped position) and have time for uninterrupted concentration. Allow yourself at least ten minutes, if possible completely alone.

Prop the book open on a table at a distance you can comfortably read. Find a chair with an upright back in which you can sit easily, facing the book; your back and shoulders should be supported, your knees slightly apart, slightly rolled outwards and feet flat on the ground. If you have short legs put your feet on a stool or otherwise raise them so that you can completely release the tension in the legs. Let your arms hang loosely with your hands on your lap. Now read through and follow the instructions slowly.

Remember to keep breathing easily and regularly throughout.

Start at the forehead Wrinkle up the skin and frown between the eyebrows . . . hold it . . . let go and release . . . frown more deeply causing deep wrinkles . . . hold it . . . let go and release . . . now frown hard, involve the whole scalp, feel the tightness . . . hold hard . . . release completely, feel the tension in the scalp relax.

Now for the eyes Screw them up just slightly, feel the wrinkles at the sides . . . hold it . . . let go and release. Screw them up more tightly until there is only a pinprick of light . . . hold . . . and release. Screw them up tightly until the nose and forehead are involved . . . hold hard . . . let go completely.

On to the mouth Pull sideways slightly . . . feel the tension . . . release. Pull the mouth into a smile . . . hold it . . . let go and release completely. Draw the mouth into a grimace . . . hold it hard . . . let go and relax.

Now the jaw Clench the teeth together . . . now release. Clench the teeth and the jaw very tightly . . . feel the tension . . . release completely so that the jaw drops, the mouth opens, and the tongue falls back.

Next the shoulders Lift slightly, hold . . . now drop. Raise the shoulders higher . . . hold them . . . release and let them fall back. Lift the shoulders to the ears . . . hold hard, let them go and feel the tension release.

Onto the hands Clench the hands into a fist and feel your fingernails in the palm . . . hold . . . and release. Clench the hands hard until the knuckles show white and you feel the tension in the shoulders . . . hold hard . . . let go and feel the tension release.

Now your trunk Push the small of your back into the chair and feel the abdomen tighten and your pelvis move . . . hold . . . and release. Repeat, making the movement stronger . . . hold longer . . . completely let go and feel yourself sink into the chair.

Down to your feet Push your heels into the ground, feel the tension in the calves and thighs . . . hold . . . let go. Press down hard . . . hold tight . . . release completely.

Continue to sit for a moment concentrating on breathing in and expanding holding the breath briefly and then expelling as a release.

When you have mastered the commands and responses, it might help to lie down in warmth and comfort (a pillow under your neck and knees if you wish) and at the start:

- Lift your head and look at your toes . . . feel the tension and release . . . repeat.
- Start at the toes and tighten your calves, buttocks, hands, shoulders, face, hold and release . . . repeat.
- Now close your eyes and think of nothing but yourself while you go through the routine slowly and steadily.

As you become more practised you will begin to be aware whenever your muscles are under tension and naturally tense and release them. There will also be times when you need to take the actions deliberately and that is when you will be really amazed at the results such as a clear mind, quicker thought and the ability to master tricky situations; this is a life enhancing skill.

SECTION 4

LIFE STYLE

Although we have put this section fourth and do not include it in the first six weeks of our Slimnastics Programme this is not because it is any less vital than the other sections in our circle. Some of the tasks set out under this section are not so simple or straightforward as the positive 'doing' of the exercises, the cooking and eating of the healthy foods and the learning and practising of the tension control technique. Now we are suggesting you make more fundamental changes in your habits which may be more difficult to tackle.

A recent television programme was called 'Consider Yourself' and perhaps self consideration is really the appropriate title for this section. For instance we believe that if time is used well it can be an aid to tension control and relaxation. However using time to our own advantage needs planning and forethought: this is not to say that we are advocating a completely disciplined, formal or restricted format for living. Although this is often the easier option at first and may seem less demanding or challenging, we can become so hidebound by our own rigidity that it can in its turn become a stress. It sometimes takes all our self-control and will-power to encourage us to break out of our old routine and living pattern. We may fear it will leave us feeling vulnerable and disorientated. However if we brave the freedom it can add up to a more fulfilled, exciting and relaxing life style with more time to care for ourselves and other people.

Both the actions of eating too much and drinking in excess can become a form of self punishment. If you give yourself some consideration and control your weight and alcohol consumption, you will in turn gain more energy to cope with the rigours of life. Giving up smoking is not only caring for yourself but also for others. Because it is so addictive you may well need expert help. You need not put on weight, you will definitely feel better and you will not regret it.

The final section is there because we feel it would be a shame once you have made such good efforts to become fit, healthy and happy only for you to get ill from food poisoning, or be maimed in an accident. We are aiming to be fit and lively not healthy but dead!

We suggest you tackle these Life Changes one by one over the weeks and only after you have really settled into the Slimnastics Programme routine. As we point out in the first part, life 'events' of this kind can be a stress in themselves.

LIFE STYLE

Use Your 'Time' Well

Break The Rules Occasionally! Every now and again it does us good to break out and 'do our own thing'. Even healthy regimes should be opted out of occasionally. This may have the benefit of really driving home the message – the physical effects from the indulgences are quickly felt for instance and the once 'oh so mouthwatering' chocolate cake becomes actually sickly! Allow yourself a day off now and again, build in lazy days, have lunch in the park, walk a different way to work, read a different author, take a risk, challenge yourself occasionally. New experiences can be enriching.

Use Your Free Time In the first place make sure you have some. It can be so much easier to continue working whether it be in the home, office, factory or at just living, than to stop and change course for a while. Hobbies, sports, evening classes, changes of scene all recharge the batteries and alleviate tensions. It is just as important to make sure these times exist as to also make sure that these extra activities themselves do not become a source of tension. It is the 'doing' which is more important than the results, it is the actual painting which is essential not the production of a masterpiece.

Seek the Company of Others It may be much easier to be on one's own and getting out of social isolation may need effort. You should also be prepared to give more than you may receive which is not easy either. However increasing social contacts can lessen stress by widening your interests, and activities done with others are usually more stress reducing than solitary ones. Meeting new people can be stimulating and rewarding. Once again, use your self control and do not expect too much of new friends but remember to value those you have known a long time. Especially do not neglect or undervalue those personal relationships which are closest to you such as husband/wife, parent/child or close friend. Much mutual support can be achieved through those who know and accept each other over the years 'warts and all'.

Enjoy some sport It takes some self-control to make time for and give energy towards some sporting activity, but physical activity is almost a necessity not only for getting fit but also for the release of nervous tension. However when the sport ceases to be fun and your ambition and drive are all directed towards 'winning' and 'succeeding' the action becomes self defeating and the sport a stress in itself. Swimming, jogging, cycling and walking are all non-competitive sports but even then you can set your own goals and carry on despite all setbacks. This is when your self-control needs to keep you in check and you will realise that in this case 'winning' is *not* coming out on top.

Take Holidays as they can lend perspective to problems and release the inhibitions. However even these breaks need some self-control. It is easy to get carried away by the brochures or other people's stories of fantastic escapades and forget that you are bored just lying in the sun, have difficulty climbing up hills, want to get away from people or need company. Choose your holidays that suit yourself and that you are capable of enjoying. Try to ensure that the break is a relaxing, regenerative and refreshing experience and not a stress in itself.

Be Flexible It is a temptation to carry on with a pre-arranged programme come what may. There are however many occasions where the force of circumstances or the necessities of the moment are such that a different arrangement is desirable or even inevitable. This is the time when you need to exercise your self-control and let go, become flexible and allow changes to be made even to the most carefully conceived plans. Try not to waste emotion on regrets but take up the new challenge with enthusiasm.

Give Yourself Space Being alone does not automatically correspond to being 'lonely', equally being surrounded by others does not always mean you feel overcrowded or hemmed in. It is useful to cultivate the art of 'switching off' or daydreaming, watching, appreciating, idling. Travelling to work, having a bath, visiting the loo, waiting at the check-out desk are all times which can be valuably used. Once more this needs some self consideration not only to take the time out from days filled with a demanding multiplicity of tasks but also to confine the time and make these times moments to treasure and not an indulgence.

Value Yourself and do not strive too long to get too far. Recognise your own worth and appreciate your successes. Exercise that control and be realistic. You are much more likely to achieve your goals if they are set at the right level for you. Constantly striving to fulfil unlikely ambitions or unfavourably comparing yourself with family, friends or rivals is unrewarding and stressful. If you know you have done well (for yourself) be pleased and if others praise you enjoy it. However remember what a boost this is to your own morale and try to look for ways in which you can applaud others too.

Be Prepared! Some 'Life Events' cannot be planned or avoided whilst others are of our own making. Attempts have been made to list Life Events in the order of the severity of their stressful impact. Death of one's spouse is usually ranked first, followed by divorce and marital separation, imprisonment, and death of a close relative (especially a parent or child). Next come personal injury and illness, loss of employment or retirement, acute sex difficulties and change in health of a family member. Even happy events such as marriage, going on holiday, Christmas, a wanted pregnancy or birth of a child have a stressful impact. The trouble starts when several life events hit you at once. There is a finite number of changes that any individual can handle at any one time. Therefore it makes sense to consider yourself when some predictable Life Event is in sight and, if possible, avoid introducing several additional changes at the same time – such as changing your job, or buying a house just when you expect a new baby to be born. Giving up smoking for instance can be a major stress and it would be a mistake to start when recently bereaved or divorced or maybe even tackling a weight problem.

Control Your Weight

This is the time for complete honesty with yourself. Are you overweight?

- Do your clothes still fit easily?
- Look at yourself naked in the mirror, at your body profile, any bulges, any changes?
- Pinch the upper arm, thigh or midriff. There should not be more than an inch of flesh between the thumb and forefinger.
- Check your recommended weight against your height.

You will see from the chart overleaf that there is quite a large margin. This is because there are several factors besides your height which influence your weight such as your sex, age, frame size, hormonal activity, diets and exercise level. If you have changed the way you are eating and your weight is still outside the range given for your height you will need to cut down your calorie intake and increase your energy output.

However, if you are obese (see the following tables) you would be very wise to take a more drastic approach; obesity should be taken very seriously.

The D.H.S.S. document 'Eating for Health' states 'Obesity is probably the most common nutritional disorder in Britain today and is an important medical problem. Not only is the expectation of life shortened but there is also an increased morbidity and mortality from certain diseases. These diseases are disabling for those affected by them and costly to the nation both in treatment and in loss of work-efficiency!

It is the food intake exceeding the energy expenditure which adds on the weight (for instance one ounce of chocolate or one pint of beer a day over the required number of calories can add up to an excess weight of 20lb (5.0kg) in a year). To lose the weight not only must the input be less than the output but also the energy expenditure must be gradually increased to ensure that the metabolism does not slow down to accommodate the decrease of energy consumption which could result in the weight loss stopping and staying at a constant level.

The increased medical risks or contributory factors of being overweight include:

- Respiratory disease
- High blood pressure
- Surgical risks
- Reduced life expectancy
- Hernias
- Varicose veins
- Heart disease
- Atherosclerosis
- Diabetes
- Inflammation of the gall bladder
- Arthritis
- Conception and pregnancy problems

Body changes in the obese include:
- Double chin
- Drooping breasts
- Fatty thighs
- Poor posture
- Flabby upper arms
- Bulging stomach
- Flat feet
- Back strain

Social problems for the obese can be:
- Clumsiness
- Perspiration
- Unsightly clothing
- Increased proneness to accidents
- Loss of attraction to others and themselves
- Higher insurance premiums

Personal effects can be:
- Unhappiness
- Tension
- Anxiety
- Lack of confidence which in turn can encourage more over eating.

It is important to remember that most children put on weight and are fatter at the beginning of adolescence, and that they will naturally take more food during this normal spurt in growth. So extra weight on children at this time is not necessarily something to worry about – the extra fat will usually have gone by the time they reach adulthood. If however they are very fat they may become fat adults, so seek expert help. It is not usually so necessary to worry about the weight and measurements of the young teenager as to make sure they have a healthy diet, a good amount of exercise and also adequate relaxation.

Losing that Excess Weight!

This may not call for as much self discipline and control as you may fear! We do *not* recommend that you should go on a rigid diet or eat slimming foods, go on some special treatment or indulge in binges or starvation. It is much better for your health to make changes which will become a permanent part of your eating habits. **If you do the following you should have no need for the above:**

Reduce your fat intake Watch out for hidden fats (in processed or tinned foods), reduce added fats and check cooking methods.

Eat no extra sugar or sugar-containing foods (or drinks) this cuts out all those unnecessary calories.

Eat more fruit and vegetables which are bulky, filling and low in fat and high in fibre and small amounts of energy may also be passed in the stools.

Change your thoughts on protein Your substitution of animal protein by vegetable protein will cut down your fat (energy) intake still further

Eat a variety of foods that will provide all the vitamins and minerals you need for your metabolism to function properly.

Read the labels on convenience foods so as to avoid hidden fats and sugars.

Limit your alcohol so you do not wastefully drink excess calories.

Eat breakfast to give you a good start to the day.

Watch your calories carefully.

Use a smaller plate, and eat slowly.

Do not nibble between meals (do not *buy* nibbles to eat!)

Make every meal an occasion even if you are only having a sandwich. Sit down and eat it on a plate with a knife and fork (if we are eating 'on the run' we can consume quantities of food without even realising that it has passed our lips – think of the sweets you can eat on a journey and still be ready for your meal on arrival).

Two other points will also help:

If you are addicted to a food try eating it very, very slowly (chewing each small mouthful say at least 20 times). This can be very disconcerting. Experiment with eating one square of chocolate in this way.

Remember that to lose weight not only must the input be less than the output but also the energy expenditure must be gradually increased to ensure that the metabolism does not slow down to accommodate the decrease of energy consumption which could result in the weight loss stopping and staying at a constant level. You will need to step up the amount of exercise you take. If you are very overweight you should not do weight bearing exercises because your joints and posture will be affected. Swimming is the best form of vigorous exercise to do alongside the Slimnastics Programme. You will need to consistently increase the length of time you are moving as well as the energy you expend.

NB Too great a weight loss is also unhealthy! Most of us are aware of the anorexic who compulsively starves him or herself or the person who alternatively binges and vomits. We know these people run the risk of malnutrition and even death in their neurotic wish to become excessively thin and their often hidden desire to delay maturity. However, it is also becoming evident that people who exercise excessively (i.e. jog obsessively, go to exercise classes continually, some people who compete in athletics), without complimentary food intake can lose so much body fat as to fall below the Body Mass Index. This states that the body weight should be between 20-25 when you put $\frac{\text{the weight (in kg)}}{\text{height (in metres}^2\text{)}}$ to be normal. Below this (19 and below) is too thin and menstruation in women may stop. Also babies born to women in this category are likely to be small and also have smaller brains. The births too may be difficult.

If all else fails do not despair. Go to your doctor, a dietician, a Slimnastics or reputable exercise class. But do not just sit there – do something! However, **beware** of 'crash' diets – they are unhealthy for the ordinary individual.

LIFE STYLE

METRIC **NON-METRIC**

The table below shows the Acceptable Average weight for both men and women relative to their height, also the Acceptable Weight Range and the weights for obesity.

	MEN			WOMEN		
Height without shoes	Acceptable Average weight	Acceptable weight range	Obese	Acceptable Average weight	Acceptable weight range	Obese
1.48m				46.5kg	42-54kg	65kg
1.50m				47.0kg	43-55kg	66kg
1.52m				48.5kg	44-57kg	68kg
1.54m				49.5kg	44-58kg	70kg
1.56m				50.4kg	45-58kg	70kg
1.58m	55.8kg	51-64kg	77kg	51.3kg	46-59kg	71kg
1.60m	57.6kg	52-65kg	78kg	52.6kg	48-61kg	73kg
1.62m	58.6kg	53-66kg	79kg	54.0kg	49-62kg	74kg
1.64m	59.6kg	54-67kg	80kg	55.4kg	50-64kg	77kg
1.66m	60.6kg	55-69kg	83kg	56.8kg	51.65kg	78kg
1.68m	61.7kg	56-71kg	85kg	58.1kg	52-66kg	79kg
1.70m	63.5kg	58-73kg	88kg	60.6kg	53-67kg	80kg
1.72m	65.0kg	59-74kg	89kg	61.3kg	55-69kg	83kg
1.74m	66.5kg	60-75kg	90kg	62.6kg	56-70kg	84kg
1.76m	68.0kg	62-77kg	92kg	64.0kg	58-72kg	86kg
1.78m	69.4kg	64-79kg	95kg			
1.80m	71.0kg	65.80kg	96kg			
1.82m	72.6kg	66-82kg	98kg			
1.84m	74.2kg	67-84kg	101kg			

	MEN			WOMEN		
Height without shoes	Acceptable average weight	Acceptable weight range	Obese	Acceptable average weight	Acceptable weight range	Obese
4'10"				7st 3lb	6st 6lb- 8st 5lb	10st 2lb
4'11"				7st 4lb	6st 7lb- 8st 7lb	10st 4lb
5'				7st 6lb	6st 9lb- 8st 9lb	10st 7lb
5' 1"				7st 9lb	7st 1lb- 9st 1lb	11st
5' 2"				8st 1lb	7st 3lb- 9st 4lb	11st
5' 3"	9st 1lb	8st 2lb-10st 3lb	12st 4lb	8st 2lb	7st 4lb- 9st 6lb	11st 5lb
5' 4"	9st 3lb	8st 4lb-10st 6lb	12st 7lb	8st 6lb	7st 7lb- 9st 9lb	11st 6lb
5' 5"	9st 5lb	8st 6lb-10st 9lb	13st	8st 8lb	7st 9lb-10st 1lb	12st 1lb
5' 6"	9st 7lb	8st 9lb-11st 1lb	13st 4lb	9st 1lb	8st 1lb-10st 4lb	12st 5lb
5' 7"	10st	9st 1lb-11st 5lb	13st 8lb	9st 4lb	8st 4lb-10st 7lb	12st 6lb
5' 8"	10st 3lb	9st 4lb-11st 9lb	14st 2lb	9st 7lb	8st 7lb-11st	13st 2lb
5' 9"	10st 6lb	9st 7lb-12st 1lb	14st 6lb	10st	9st -11st 3lb	13st 6lb
5'10"	10st 9lb	10st -12st 4lb	14st 9lb	10st 3lb	9st 3lb-11st 6lb	14st
5'11"	11st 3lb	10st 3lb-12st 8lb	15st 4lb	10st 6lb	9st 6lb-12st	14st 4lb
6'	11st 6lb	10st 6lb-13st 1lb	15st 8lb	10st 8lb	9st 8lb-12st 4lb	14st 6lb
6' 1"	11st 9lb	10st 9lb-13st 5lb	16st 2lb			
6' 2"	12st 2lb	11st 1lb-13st 9lb	16st 6lb			
6' 3"	12st 6lb	11st 4lb-14st 2lb	17st			
6' 4"	12st 9lb	11st 7lb-14st 6lb	17st 5lb			

Limit that Alcohol

Most of us enjoy a drink; it is a social habit, revives the spirit, lifts the soul, loosens the tongue and enhances good food. We associate alcohol with celebrations, free time, relaxation, get-togethers and general *bonhomie*. It is easy to see how you can fall into the trap of using its effects when you feel lonely, depressed, inadequate or just overworked.

Nearly everyone can now buy alcohol simply and discreetly through their local supermarket and the proportion of alcohol in the diet has doubled since the 1950s. It now represents 4-9% of the daily food energy intake of the population. There is a marked increase in the alcoholic consumption of women and youngsters and this continues to rise.

Much of the nation's excess weight may be caused through regular alcoholic intake by people who are already eating an adequate diet; and for some people it is the opposite, with drink taking the place of a good varied diet and resulting in malnutrition. However, your weight may not be your only problem when you do not limit your alcohol; you have only to glance down the results potentially suffered by the 'Accept' man (see illustration opposite) to understand that the health hazards of alcohol should not be underestimated.

Behaviour Problems

Alcohol is a narcotic and anaesthetic. It numbs the brain and the Central Nervous System, having the same effect as morphine or chloroform . . . it is not surprising that under its influence accidents can occur.

Alcohol is a primary and continuous depressant slowing down the workings of the brain. It depresses the part of the brain which controls behaviour, and impairs the senses and the ability to judge and react to situations. A person may appear to be more sociable and talkative . . . what is actually happening is that their potential ability to make rational thought-out decisions is being impaired.

Social Results

Road Accidents In 1974 35% of all drivers who died in road accidents had been drinking (Blennerhassett Report 1976).

Accidents at Work The cost to British industry through drinking problems is estimated to be getting close to £350 million; 3 times as many people with a drinking problem are involved in accidents at work than are others, and similarly they lose 2 to 3 times as many working days through sickness (Report of the Working Party on Alcohol and Work, NCA 1979).

Crime 89% of heavy drinkers in prison claimed alcohol had played an important part in causing their latest crime (Manle & Cooper 1966).

Family and Home Drinking habits can

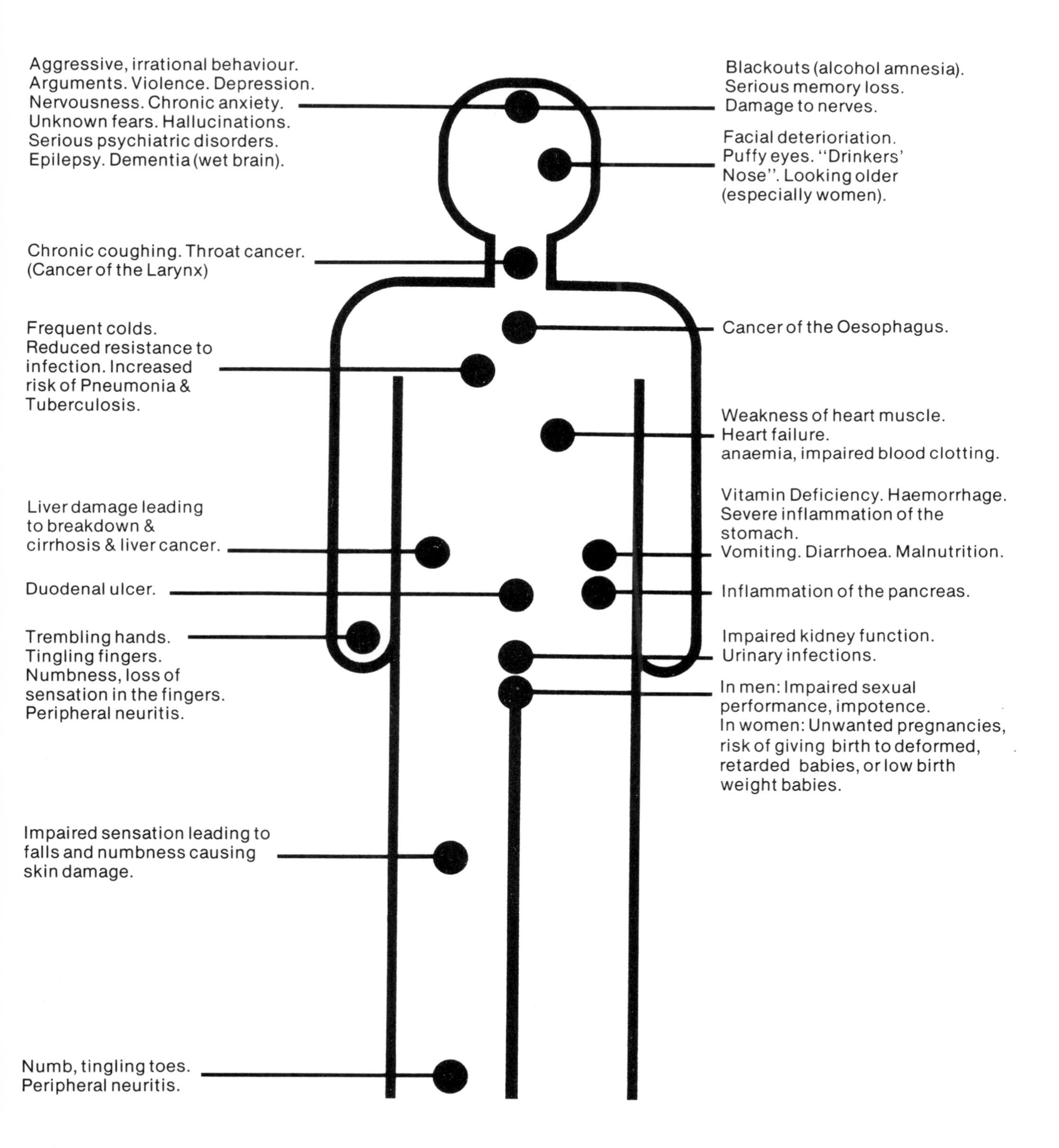
Aggressive, irrational behaviour.
Arguments. Violence. Depression.
Nervousness. Chronic anxiety.
Unknown fears. Hallucinations.
Serious psychiatric disorders.
Epilepsy. Dementia (wet brain).
Blackouts (alcohol amnesia).
Serious memory loss.
Damage to nerves.
Facial deterioriation.
Puffy eyes. "Drinkers' Nose". Looking older (especially women).
Chronic coughing. Throat cancer. (Cancer of the Larynx)
Cancer of the Oesophagus.
Frequent colds. Reduced resistance to infection. Increased risk of Pneumonia & Tuberculosis.
Weakness of heart muscle.
Heart failure.
anaemia, impaired blood clotting.
Vitamin Deficiency. Haemorrhage.
Severe inflammation of the stomach.
Vomiting. Diarrhoea. Malnutrition.
Liver damage leading to breakdown & cirrhosis & liver cancer.
Duodenal ulcer.
Inflammation of the pancreas.
Trembling hands.
Tingling fingers.
Numbness, loss of sensation in the fingers.
Peripheral neuritis.
Impaired kidney function.
Urinary infections.
In men: Impaired sexual performance, impotence.
In women: Unwanted pregnancies, risk of giving birth to deformed, retarded babies, or low birth weight babies.
Impaired sensation leading to falls and numbness causing skin damage.
Numb, tingling toes.
Peripheral neuritis.

affect relationships and social behaviour especially with family and friends. Eventually a person can become so dependent physically and psychologically as to be called an alcoholic. Drinking during pregnancy can affect or harm the unborn child.

Hospital Admissions Because of accidents or illness alcohol is very expensive for the country.

Health Problems

As a source of energy, alcohol is useless; it can retard body growth and maintenance, it does not repair tissues, it hinders an absorption of some vitamins and minerals, it is unable to be stored in the body and it causes loss of body heat and dehydration and lowers the resistance to infection.

Without oxygen all cells will die. Diseases like malaria, cancer and syphillis cause the red blood cells to become sticky and sluggish so that they are unable to move through the tiny blood vessels called capillaries and deliver the vital oxygen in time. Alcohol causes the same thing to happen; many cells become damaged and die.

Alcohol enlarges the blood vessels and therefore increases the skin temperature. This causes loss of body heat and chilling although giving a false feeling of extra warmth. Antarctic explorers and mountaineers are well aware of the dangers of this.

Excessive drinking can contribute to illnesses in the:

Liver which can become fatty then scarred and diseased (cirrhosis). Death rates due to this are steadily rising.

Stomach where there can be inflammation which can be a factor in the formation of peptic ulcers (it also slows down the rate of healing).

Heart which can become fatty; the muscles can also become weakened contributing to heart failure.

Nervous System which can degenerate and the brain be damaged.

How Much is Too Much?

1 unit of alcohol = ½ pint beer / 1 glass of table wine / 1 glass sherry / 1 single whisky (pub measure).

Effect on the Body

2 units likelihood of accidents begins to increase.

3 units you feel more cheerful, feeling of warmth. Impaired judgement and inhibition.

5 units loss of driving licence.

10 units loss of self-control, exuberance, quarrelsome, slurred speech.

13 units stagger, double vision, loss of memory.

¾ bottle of spirits oblivion, sleepiness, coma.

More than 1 bottle of spirits death possible.

You are considered over the limit for driving if you have had 5 units or more. Large doses kill by arresting breathing. Often unconsciousness occurs before this stage. What is a safe level for you? It is difficult to say as everyone differs greatly, although over 6 units a day for men and 3 for women is known to be above the danger level.

Alcohol and You

The facts above must prove that excess alcohol and health do not go together. It makes good sense to limit your alcohol intake; unfortunately as the table above shows, after three measures good sense may well be overruled by the effect of the drink. Because of this it is essential to set yourself limits before you *start* to drink and really convince yourself that to take any more will do you actual physical harm.

Stick to your pre-thought-out number of measures.

Dilute your drink with low-calorie mixer or mineral water, it will last longer that way.

Alternate alcoholic drinks with non-alcoholic ones.

Never drink straight spirits – they are more easily absorbed into the blood stream.

Never drink alone – that can lead to a slippery path!

Always respect alcohol – in small amounts it is a pleasure; in excess it spells trouble.

Be a good host and provide alternative drinks and respect others when they want to cut down.

Make sure alcoholic drinks do not replace meals.

Remember that alcohol can be just as high in calories as some solid foods. Be aware if you are watching your weight that the more you drink the less likely you are to worry about what you eat!

Smoking is a DANGEROUS Habit!

So far in this book we have been concentrating on the positive actions we can take to help ourselves get and stay as healthy as possible. Now however we have come to a definite negative for a truly healthy existence – smoking. Smoking tobacco is a deadly habit – it will either cause us to die long before our appointed time or may lead to us enduring a living death. There is a story which may be apocryphal but which illustrates the seriousness with which we should regard the habit: the natives, upset by the behaviour of Sir Walter Raleigh and his men when they plundered the Americas on behalf of the first Queen Elizabeth, took a cunning revenge. Sir Walter on the lookout for exciting trophies to take back to his Monarch asked to be shown the plants the leaves of which seemed to give so much pleasure to those who were rolling, lighting and inhaling the smoke. He was directed to fields in which grew two different plants – he was given the plant called nicotene, the other was called marajuana. In fact the nicotene was used as an insecticide and is still used as such very effectively in the present day. It is a lethal poison.

Why do we do this to ourselves despite the fact that most of us are aware of the dangers? Why are the numbers of smokers not decreasing? The latest report on 'Smoking among Secondary School Children' shows that nearly £60 million worth of cigarettes are smoked a year by children aged between 11 and 16. We have to face the fact that it pays countries, governments, importers and manufacturers to keep the tobacco industry flourishing. Advertising, image making and many other subtle forces make smoking an attractive and exciting act and after that the nicotene can take over by itself – it is an alkaloid drug and has very powerful effects on the nervous system and heart. There is also a rumour that countries and governments could not afford to allow us to 'kick the habit' – we might become such healthy, long lived nations that the expense of the larger active population would be too great!

It is therefore up to us personally to help ourselves. It is constantly said that it is very difficult to give it up. However this is belied by the heart patients who stop abruptly, and simply have no urge at all to start again. Indeed they care so much about living that just to meet a few of them might be enough for some of us to throw the packet away. Anyone who has had a coronary actually believes, knows completely, that smoking is an obnoxious habit and does nothing but harm. This belief is so complete that they would no more touch a cigarette than pick and eat the plant deadly nightshade.

What is in a Cigarette?

Nicotene is an alkaloid drug and one of the most powerful poisons known. The average smoker absorbs 2 milligrams of nicotene from a cigarette. There seems little doubt that it is nocotene which is the habit-forming drug in smoking. Medical tests when nicotene injections have been given to smokers result in less cigarettes being smoked. Effects of nicotene on the body are:

- To cause the surface blood vessels of the limbs to constrict.
- It raises the blood pressure and speeds up the heart rate therefore making more blood leave the heart faster.
- It impairs the absorption of vitamin C, and some researchers believe it also destroys the vitamin C already present in the blood (25mg of vitamin C is needed to replace that lost by smoking just one cigarette).
- It constricts the blood vessels of the mouth and prevents the phagocytes (the body's first line of defence against bacterial invasion) from working and this increases the chance of infection. It has been established that one cigarette puts this part of the defence mechanism out of action for 15 minutes.

Carbon Monoxide reduces the flow of oxygen to the heart making any form of exercise more difficult (smoke inhaled contains 5% carbon monoxide).

Hydrogen Cyanide is also inhaled. This is a powerful poison which is present in quantities 160 times those considered safe in industry.

Phenol is also present. This is a corrosive poison and a severe irritant used to make paint and plastics.

Other Chemicals Cigarette smoke contains hundreds of different chemicals many of which are known to cause cancer in animals.

- Appreciable quantities of these compounds are inhaled with the smoke and may be the cause of cancer.
- They also act as cancer promoters which cause and encourage cancers to grow more quickly once it has started.

Other Substances narrow the bronchial tubes causing coughing and wheezing, and make breathing more difficult. They also paralyse the cilia (minute hairs which keep the lungs clean by sweeping up inhaled debris) leaving the lungs more prone to infection or tumour.

Surely there can be no good reason for deliberately allowing these substances to invade your body!

Effects of Smoking on the Body (Everyday effects)

It is unattractive. There is a lingering smell on the clothes, hands and hair; staining of nicotene on fingers and teeth and a 'bad' taste remaining in the mouth.

An impaired athletic performance – oxygen is transferred less efficiently to the muscles by the lungs. These muscles include the heart.

Sinus trouble, chest infections, lingering colds 30 million working days are lost each year through smoking-related problems.

The early morning smoker's cough – there is present in the smoke of a cigarette a chemical called benzpyrene which has the effect of paralysing the normal cough reflex which would result in response to hot smoke being breathed into the lungs. In the morning before the first cigarette, this reflex is functioning again and the hacking and spitting characteristic of the 'smoker's cough' will go on until a new dose of benzpyrene has been sucked in.

Coughing can be the first sign of damage to throat and lungs. This can lead to bronchitis. Damage to the lungs stops when smoking ceases and it may even begin to heal. There is sometimes permanent loss of use leaving a person breathless all his life.

More Serious Effects

Lung Cancer As yet research has not shown positively the causes of cancer (i.e. why cells change their normal rate of regular growth, multiplying rapidly and spreading through the body destroying and invading other tissues) however there is conclusive evidence that smoking cigarettes increases the liability of the cells in the bronchial tubes to undergo this malignant change.

- The death rate from lung cancer in the heavy smoker is 20 to 30 times greater than among non-smokers. 95% of lung cancer patients are smokers and 70% smoke more than 20 a day. The chance of getting lung cancer increases dramatically as the rate of smoking goes up. In smokers the rate is up to 1 in 8; in non-smokers it is 1:220 approx.

Chronic Bronchitis Heavy smokers are 5 times more likely to be admitted to hospital with this disease than non-smokers. The continuous irritation caused by the smoke can lead to a narrowing of the tubes so that it becomes increasingly difficult to breathe. Chronic bronchitis is one of the most common seriously disabling and killing diseases in Great Britain and it almost never occurs in non-smokers.

Coronary Heart Disease There is no definite proof but a strong suspicion that cigarette smoking increases the risk of dying from heart disease. Together with other facts such as high blood pressure, high levels of cholesterol, obesity, lack of exercise and heredity, smoking plays a major part in coronary heart disease. People who smoke one packet of cigarettes per day are twice as likely to die from a coronary as non-smokers.

Smoking is indicated in other diseases

Cancer of the mouth, throat, gullet and bladder.

Ulcers, gastric and duodenal symptoms are increased and their rate of healing is slower.

Arteries can be seriously damaged in the body and legs. This can result in the narrower arteries supplying less blood and in the legs this can make walking very painful.

Shorter life expectancy 4 out of 10 men aged 35 who smoke 25 + a day will not reach 65; 6 out of 7 non-smokers will. The Royal College of Physicians calculate that on average a smoker loses 5½ minutes of his life for each cigarette smoked.

The Effects on Others

Pregnancy

- Smoking affects the growth rate of the baby which on average may be 8oz lighter than normal.
- Nicotene and carbon monoxide with the other chemicals are carried via the blood, womb and placenta to the baby's circulation depriving the baby's tissues of oxygen.
- Smoking after the fourth month of pregnancy can lead to stillbirth or a cot death.

Small Children

- breathe in germs from their parents cough, and air which is polluted by the smoke is directly damaging to their lungs.
- Babies with smoking parents are more prone to pneumonia and bronchitis in the first year of life and chest infections in their early years.

LIFE STYLE

Smoking Homes!

- Lung cancer among non-smokers who live or are constantly with heavy smokers is twice as high as those who live in a non-smoking atmosphere. Non-smoking spouses married to heavy smokers die on average 4 times earlier than those married to non-smokers.

Giving Up the 'Odious Weed'

By now, if you have allowed yourself to get this far, you must be convinced that smoking is not good for your health. But how are you going to give it up? First of all, you must believe to your very inmost being that smoking is harmful.

Now, pick your time Try to avoid giving up smoking during times of obvious stress such as Christmas. Pick a period of already altered timetable such as a holiday or after an illness such as 'flu, or a time when you are busy but under no particular strain.

Alter your routine deliberately so that you do not meet the usual triggers which make you automatically reach for a cigarette.

Keep yourself occupied with some new and demanding activity, especially something physical so that your energies are fully extended.

Deliberately ensure you frequent non-smoking areas, in trains, buses, cinemas, etc.

Be prepared for the withdrawal symptoms which may include trembling, sweating, irritability, anxiety and insomnia; even if severe these are unlikely to last for more than 4 to 6 weeks and may disappear sooner especially if your addiction was purely a psychological one. You may want to eat more but this is only a physiological response to the previously depressed appetite and in part a replacement activity. If you stick to a healthy diet any marginal increase in weight will soon disappear.

Give yourself extra vitamins such as the B complex as they have a calming effect and also C to compensate for that which was lost.

Drink frequently to wash the toxins from the system.

Shower often massaging the body with a sponge and towelling down well. This will help the toxins to be eliminated from the pores.

Concentrate on the benefits. You will:

- Look better, feel fitter and have more money to spend.
- Have a greater resistance to many illnesses such as coughs and colds.
- Use your heart and lungs more efficiently which will give you more energy.
- Have a reduced risk of suffering from smoking-related diseases – cancer, coronaries, hypertension, etc.
- Have an increased life expectancy.

In the recent report from the Royal College of Physicians entitled 'Health on Smoking' they say 'tobacco still accounts for 15-20% of all deaths in Britain: of every 1,000 young men who smoke, one will be murdered, six will die on the roads but 250 will be killed before their time by tobacco!

If all else fails seek medical help *before* it becomes essential.

Take Care of Yourself

Learn to Take Care of Others and Yourself First Aid is often said to be simply common sense but this is a dangerous over-simplification. It is surprising that such a vital subject as First Aid should be so neglected in school curricula. It is important that you should fill this gap by taking a course yourself as soon as you are able. There are many excellent ones often taking no more than six weeks run by the Red Cross, St John's Ambulance and many Adult Colleges. They are well worth attending and you will be surprised how many times you may have to put the knowledge you will learn into operation.

Make Sure Your Home is not a Hazard
Check your lighting (any dark spots?), furniture (loose rugs), electrical appliances, fire risks and prevention, garden safety and your knowledge of the local services. Keep pinned to the wall by your telephone a notice with your name, address and telephone number on it together with the numbers of your own doctor, local police station, hospital with a Casualty Ward, plus the Emergency Call 999. This may sound as though you are being overcautious but under tension and panic every thought can disappear from your head and many a fireman is left holding the line asking patiently 'What is your address?' over and over again as the fire begins to get a hold.

Do Not Run the Risk of Accidental Poisoning

- Keep all medicines labelled correctly and out of the reach of small children. Tell the chemist if you are taking any other drugs as some medicines do not mix with others. Throw them away when the illness is over; medicines deteriorate.
- Never store poisonous substances in innocent-looking containers such as white spirit in a gin bottle. It can be lethal.
- Lavatories must be kept scrupulously clean but do not pour both bleach and a proprietary toilet cleanser down a sink or loo at the same time – poisonous chlorine gas is given off.

Hygiene in the Kitchen Makes Sense
Food poisoning causes illness and in the elderly, infants and people who have already been ill it can be positively dangerous. There are some simple precautions you can take:

- The body is a warm, comfortable place for germs so to avoid transferring them to the food make sure you and your clothes are clean.
- Always clean and cover a wound, cut or burn so these germs and bacteria too will not transfer to the food.
- Raw meat, including poultry, may be contaminated on arrival in the kitchen. Cooking can kill off dangerous germs before the food is eaten, but be careful to keep all knives and boards involved in the preparation of raw meat entirely separate from untensils used when preparing cooked meats and other foods. Cooked meat should be covered and stored above any raw meat in the same refrigerator.
- Germs hate heat, but love the warmth. Reheating food will not destroy germs unless it is thoroughly heated through sufficiently. For the same reason cooled food should always be cooked as quickly as possible.
- Chickens and other poultry must be completely unfrozen before any cooking takes place. They should then be thoroughly cooked.

Cherish Your Teeth You can do more with your mouth than just eat and speak – you can express your emotions, and reveal your personality. If your teeth are painful or ugly your whole being becomes affected. Poor teeth can also dictate the type of diet you eat even reducing you to concentrate on soft, pulpy, mashed foods which do not require biting or chewing. Eating the foods which we recommend for general health and in particular avoiding all refined sugary foods and drinks will greatly reduce the sugar-induced dental caries and gum disease. However you still need to clean your teeth thoroughly twice a day using a good toothpaste (recommended by your dentist). Dental floss is also highly recommended.

Give your hearing a chance! Disco-goers and personal hi-fi users have been warned that too much loud music can lead to deafness. This applies equally to anyone who lives or works in a noisy environment. Normally we hear sounds because tiny hair-like cells within the inner ear vibrate when sound waves hit them and turn the signal into an electrical impulse which the brain can understand. However a very loud noise or too much exposure to noise can damage and kill those cells. The problem, for those deafened by noise, is that the cells first damaged are those which pick up high frequency sounds which are important in language – sounds like ch, sh or f. A person deafened by noise, therefore, will still be able to hear low frequency background noises and be aware of conversation but will not be able to understand what is being said. This type of deafness is permanent and is extremely difficult to help with a hearing aid. Another added problem is that this kind of damage can also lead to tinnitus sometimes described as a 'ringing' in the head but more often sounding like a road drill or aeroplane taking off.

Do not Needlessly Harm Yourself: In many ways we do ourselves harm because we simply do not realise the facts:

Watch the amount of tea and coffee (especially black) which you consume. They both contain powerful stimulants which in quantity have a substantial effect on your metabolism and behaviour. If you feel 'twitchy' try changing to de-caffeinated coffee; if you feel 'windy' suspect the amount of tea you drink.

Be careful when you sunbathe. It may look healthy and fit to be tanned but over exposure to sunlight can cause more problems than it cures. It is well known that the most important skin cancer factor is sunlight exposure but it is also linked to hormone upsets, cataracts, migraines, and just plain early ageing.

Check your vitamins and minerals Although medicines can cure they also cause problems in other parts of the body. As you can see from the Vitamin and Mineral Tables, antibiotics, the contraceptive pill, and others have quite an effect on the body's absorption of these vital nutrients. It is wise to make sure you have enough vitamins and minerals as well as natural yoghurt (which replaces the bacteria) if you use these drugs.

Try the natural remedies If your medicine cabinet is full of drugs to cure the normal ailments such as headaches, pain, sore eyes, sleeplessness and so on, why not try some of the natural products which can be obtained from the Health Shops which are gentle, can be very effective and relieve a range of complaints without unpleasant side effects?

Consider Alternative Medicine Orthodox Medicine is an essential safeguard and aid for life but there are also many Alternative Medicine ideas which are worth exploring and which adopt a 'whole person' approach. None of these claim to have all the answers but they are gradually and deservedly gaining a greater public following.

Consider your sex life Remember that the safest way to avoid catching all venereal diseases is to know and trust one sexual partner. The more partners you have the more vulnerable you become. Using a sheath is a help in some cases and careful hygiene is a slight help but promiscuity is a health risk. If you do catch a sexually-transmitted disease it is essential, not only for you but also for your partners, to attend a clinic very quickly.

THE SLIMNASTICS PROGRAMME

Up to now we have concentrated on the background thinking, theories and facts about the 'whole person' approach to health and fitness. We hope we have convinced you that this is the way to get fit and that you are now ready to put it into practice. This is YOUR part of the book. We will give you the guidelines but it is up to you to put it into ACTION. We hope you will enjoy it, you will almost certainly feel better for doing it.

The Slimnastics Exercises

We have given you twelve programmes of exercises which should take only **six minutes of your time each day for 12 weeks.** Over the following 12 weeks we have suggested that you increase the time to twelve minutes a day and you can then progress to 24 minutes a day and even longer if you can spare the time and want to get really fit.

These programmes have been carefully thought out to help your body to get fit slowly but surely, without strain (but with a little pressure!), enabling you to feel good, look your best and improve your health and performance. The first figure of each exercise shows the correct starting position. The six exercises a day start with one for suppleness, to loosen and mobilise your joints using your own natural range, and go on to the vital one which will improve your stamina by more involvement of the Cardio/Vascular/Respiratory System (in other words your heart, circulation and breathing). This is followed by an exercise specifically designed to improve your shape by toning up the muscles of certain parts of the body, enabling you to look better and at the same time helping the posture and internal muscles. The fourth exercise has the emphasis on strength and the fifth concentrates on stretch and elasticity. Number six rounds the programme off with an exercise for co-ordination, skill and balance which at the same time gradually allows your body to slow down.

For the first 12 weeks the exercises should all be done for 1 minute each. The exercises progress from week to week and if you at any time find an exercise difficult, substitute it with one from the week before (or even before that if you have for instance any difficulty with kneeling). The Slimnastics exercises are not meant to be provocative (unlike some physiotherapy exercises which are used with great skill but with one-to-one monitoring, or other form of exercises which have been designed for and executed by those who are already exceptionally fit); in other words they do not attempt to push you to your limits or cause any distress. Do not be disappointed if you do not feel stiff or exhausted. Some people have the mistaken notion that this is the necessary result of a good 'work out'! This is not the case. You should in fact feel more invigorated and alert as well as relaxed when you have finished the exercises – not sweaty, tired and exhausted.

Choose a time of day which is convenient for you to have a quarter of an hour to yourself. Do not allow yourself to mislead your thoughts into being convinced that there is no time available . . . there is always time to do something you really want to do and exercising should be just as important as cleaning your teeth.

Tension Control Technique

After you have done the exercises for six minutes you will be ready to study and learn the relaxation programme and tension control technique. Make sure you are warm and comfortable and cannot be disturbed. Practise every day on your own but of course as soon as you have begun to master the programme you will be able to use it in your everyday life. However five minutes more total relaxation is worth its weight in gold as it is refreshing both mentally and physically.

The Slimnastics Healthy Eating Programme

The Weekly Programme will take you step by step towards this much healthier way of eating. Some of you may find the changes and thoughts quite revolutionary but if you truly follow the guidelines, buy the right foods, cook in the correct way and use different 'tastes' you will discover that you not only feel better and look good, your weight will most probably stabilise at an optimum level and you may well be fired with enthusiasm for different foods and tastes. It may take time, but gradually you will understand what an exciting as well as beneficial way of eating this can be.

Your Life Style

We have left the more difficult adjustments to Healthy Living until the second 12 weeks – not fearing they will be unpopular but because we are following our own advice that too many Life Events at one time is overloading the system. Taking on regular exercise, learning tension control and changing your way of eating are enough to begin with. We tackle the limiting of alcohol, giving up smoking and looking after yourself in the second part. They are essential ingredients in the Slimnastics Programme and need to be tackled one by one with some determination.

We have woven 'The Use of Your Time' into the Tension Control Programme and 'Obesity' comes naturally under the heading of Healthy Eating so you will be well on your way to a Healthy Life Style by the start of the second 12 weeks.

Before You Start

If you have any medical problems, take regular medication, have been ill or had an accident recently, suffer any permanent disabiliity, have or have had a bad back, are grossly overweight, are pregnant or had a baby during the last three months, it would be wise to check with the doctor that you are able to follow this programme. He is most likely to thoroughly approve and encourage you to start straight away but it is always sensible to make sure.

*   *   *   *

Now it is CRUNCH TIME!

It is time to meet yourself as you really are! It is difficult to be really honest with yourself but as our aim is to 'get fit' you need to know the basic material you have to work on. Fill in this form below (or trace it on to a separate sheet of paper if you don't want to write in the book) and continue to chart your progress every six weeks.

Measure yourself carefully (or ask a friend) making sure you really are honest about the bulgy bits. After all there is no point in lying to yourself especially as they are only likely to get better. Weigh on the same machine on a flat floor in the same clothes (or no clothes) at the same time of the day each time. We ask you to weigh each week but the weight loss/gain or stability will be most obvious every six weeks (remember that women invariably gain during the week of their period).

Check your weight against the Recommended Weights Chart (p. 50). Also take a good look at yourself in the mirror. Face up to reality now and then look forward to the future.

Slimnastics Individual Statistics Chart

	Week 1	Week 2	Week 3	Week 4	Week 5	Week 6
Bust						
Spare Tyre						
Waist						
Hips						
Thigh (Rt)						
Thigh (Lt)						
Upper Arm (Rt)						
Upper Arm (Lt)						
Height						
Weight						
Ideal Weight						
Weight Loss						
Measurement Loss						

THE SLIMNASTICS PROGRAMME

Week I
Healthy Eating Programme

This week eat perfectly normally but at the same time record it all on the form in the appendix (or trace it onto a separate sheet of paper). Make sure you are being completely honest (after all no one is going to benefit except yourself) and do not leave anything out.

At the end of the week ask yourself some questions:

- Is your diet high in fat? (remember the tins and processed foods).
- Is there enough fibre? (fruit, vegetables and cereals).
- Are there too many refined carbohydrates? (cakes, puddings, biscuits, etc).
- What is the salt content of your meals?
- Are you eating a varied and balanced diet but just too much of everything?

Underline the chart where you feel you could improve it.

Tension Control Technique

After you have finished the 6 minutes of exercises, put on some warmer clothes and sit down comfortably with this book. Make sure your head, neck and arms are supported, your feet are flat on the floor, your knees rolled out sideways. Breathe slowly and rhythmically. Read through the TCT on page 46 and gently follow the commands with your body. Allow at least five minutes and if you prefer, you can murmur the text out loud. It is easier to learn this way.

Weight this Week: ....st. .... lb.

The Slimnastics Exercises

Read the Safety Guidelines on page 18. Wear comfortable clothing. Barefeet or non-slip shoes.

Week 1 Do each exercise for 1 minute.

Exercise One

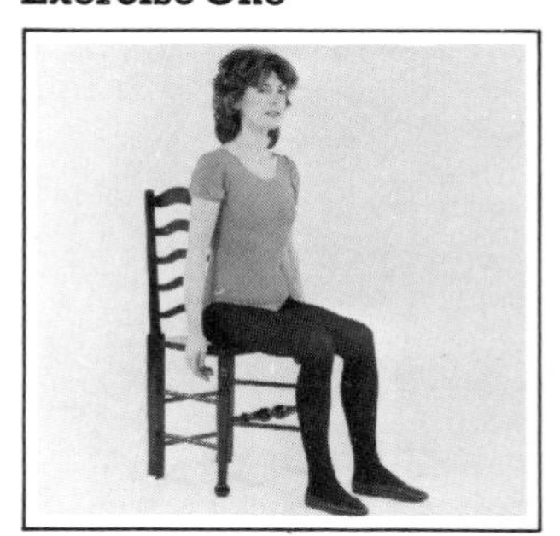

Start Sitting forward in chair. Sit tall, feet apart on floor under knees. Arms by sides. Relax and breathe easily.

▽

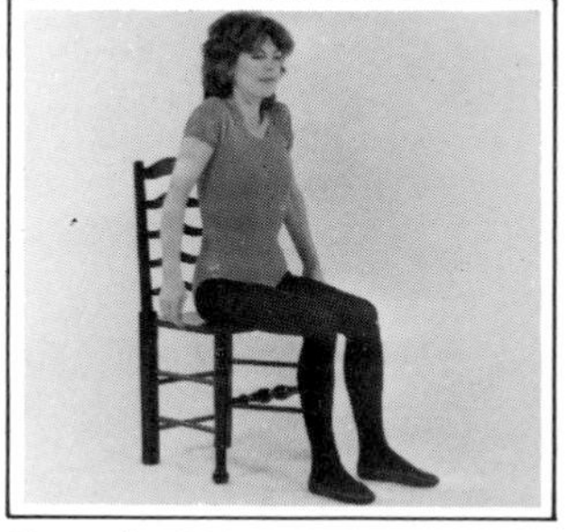

Exercise Lift shoulders up and down.
Feel Slow movement and stretched spine.

▽

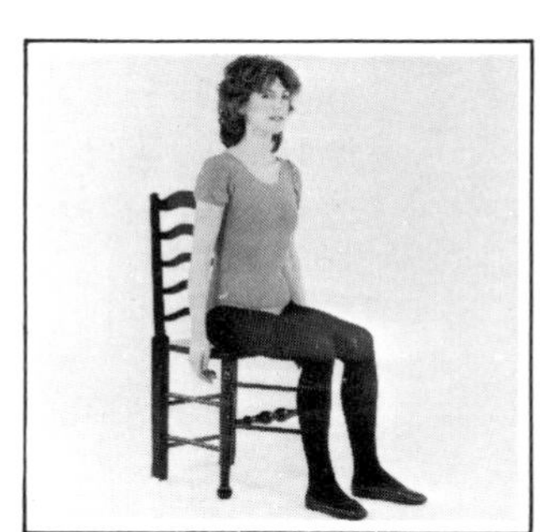

Good For Shoulders, arms, back. Relief of fatigue in shoulder area.

Exercise Two

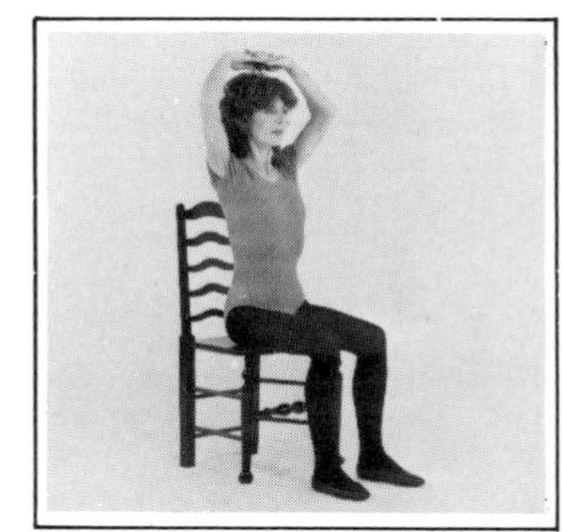

Start Sit tall. Place hands lightly above head. Feet apart.

▽

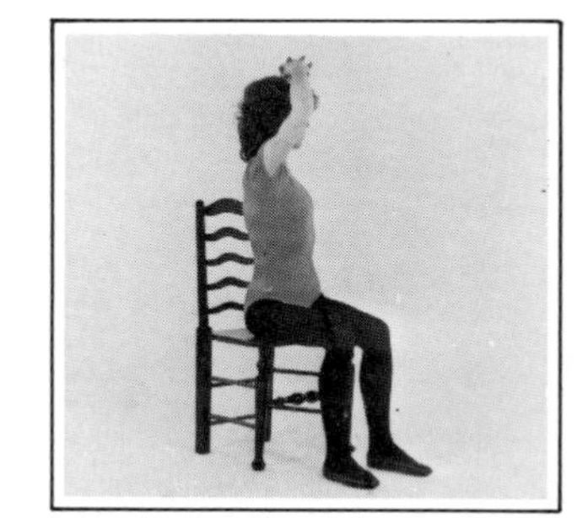

Exercise Turn trunk, one way, then the other.
Feel Firm shoulders and twisted spine.

▽

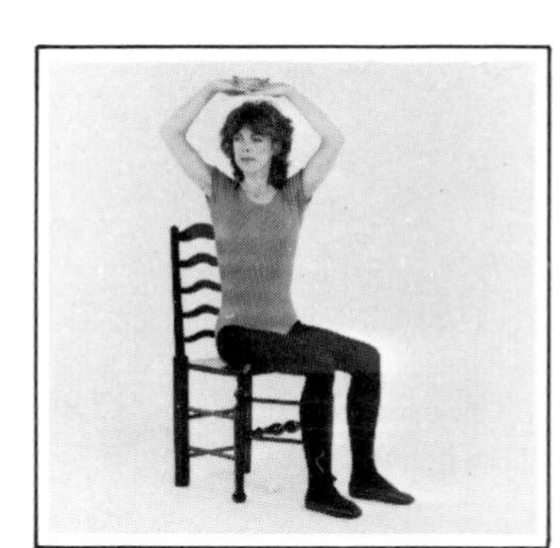

Good For Waist and spine.

WEEK 1

Exercise Three

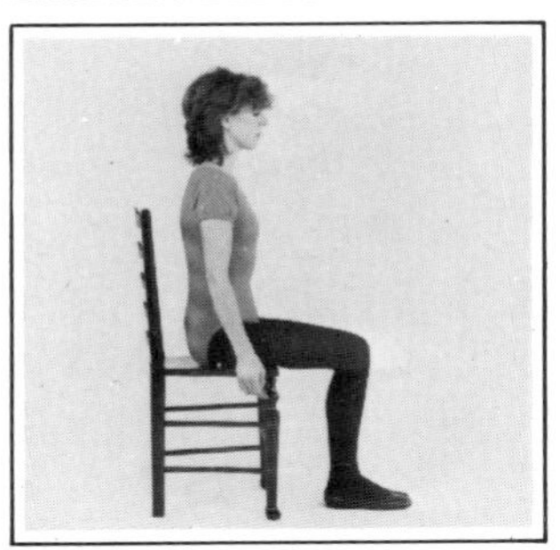

Start Sit tall, arms down by sides.
▽

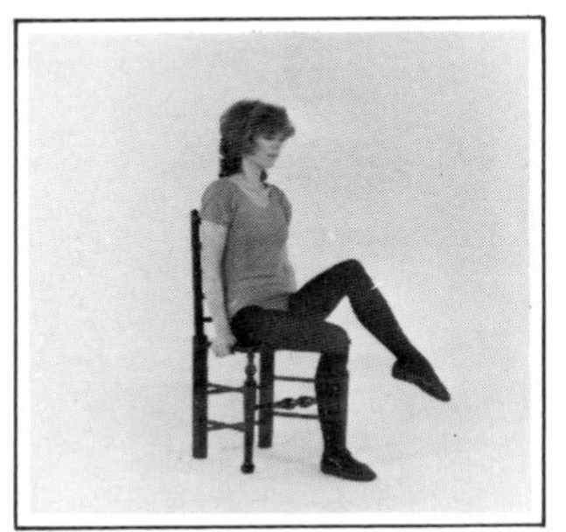

Exercise Circle ankle, change leg.
Feel Tall spine and warm feet.
▽

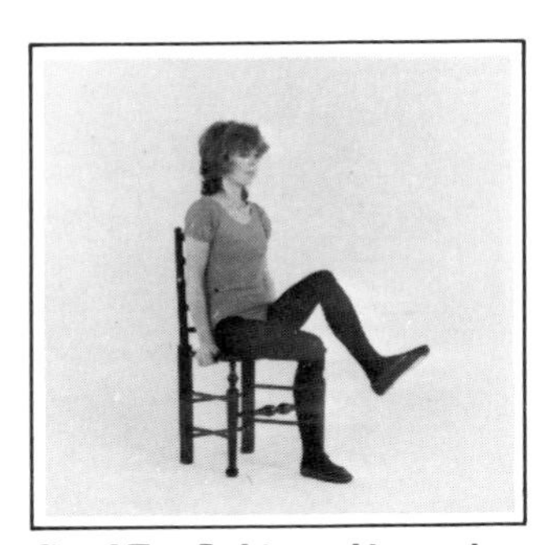

Good For Ankle and lower leg.

Exercise Four

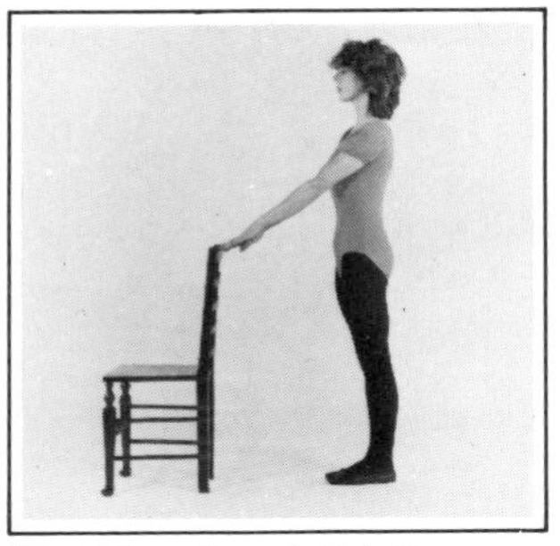

Start Place hands lightly on chair back. Stand tall, tummy and buttocks firm. Relax shoulders, breathe easily.
▽

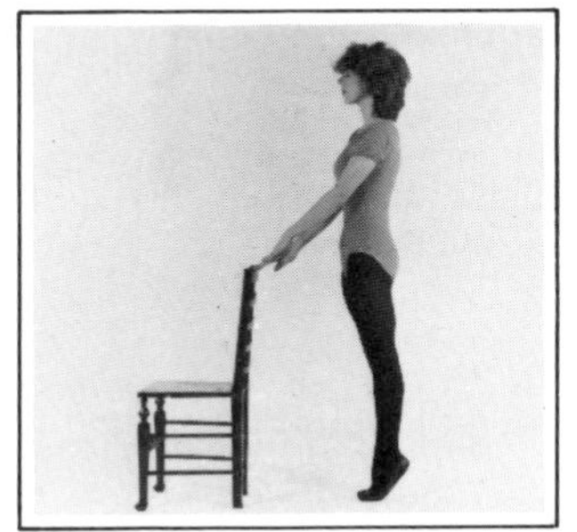

Exercise Up onto tip toes then down onto heel and lift toes off floor.
Feel Tall spine and firm body.
▽

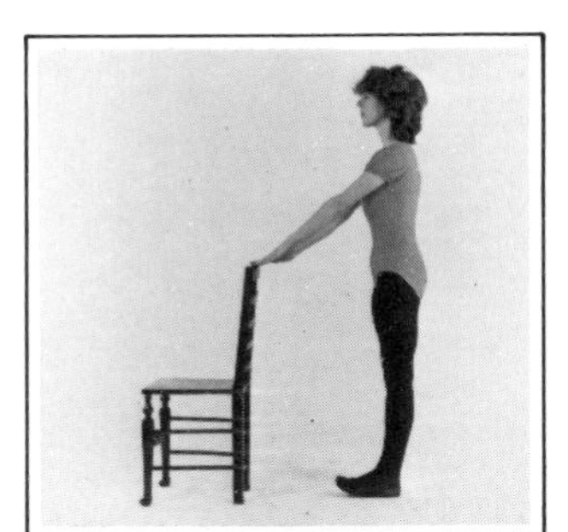

Good For Posture, legs and feet.

Exercise Five

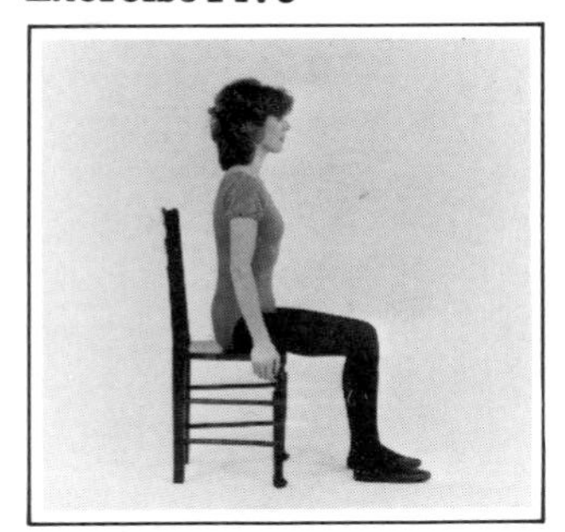

Start Sit tall.
▽

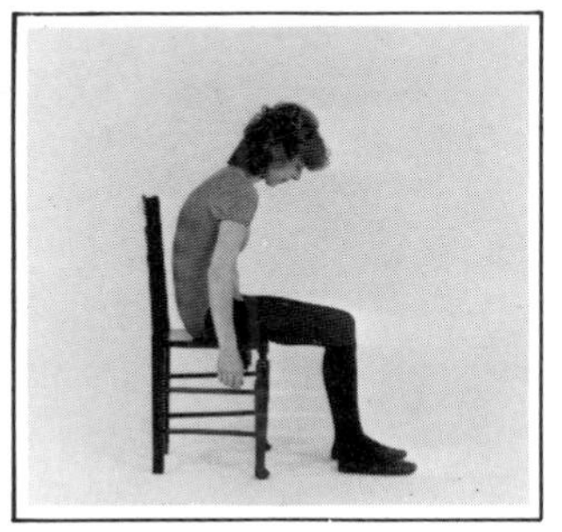

Exercise Roll pelvis backwards and round the spine with head down; then stretch the spine with head up.
Feel Round back and stretched spine.
▽

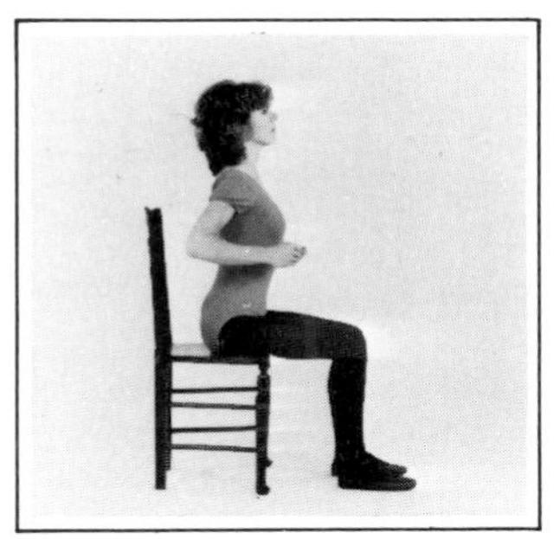

Good For Pelvis, hips, spine, pelvic tilting.

Exercise Six

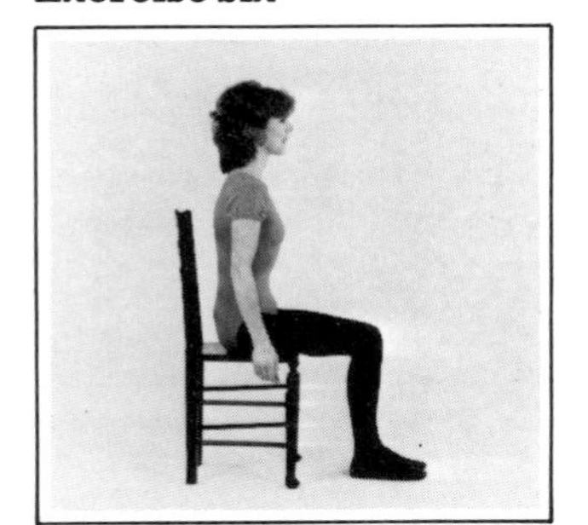

Start Sit tall, back straight, relax shoulders.
▽

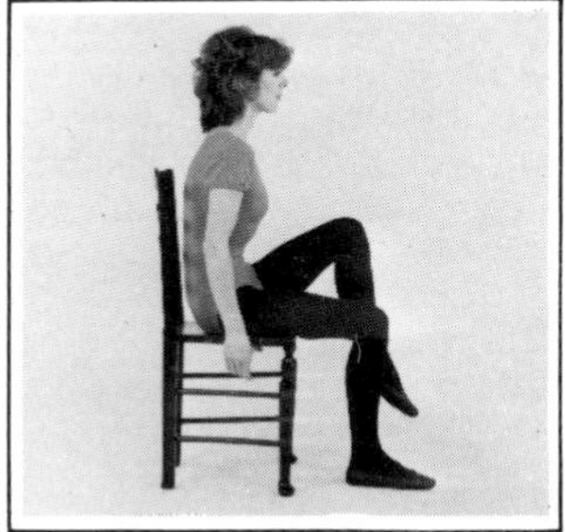

Exercise Bend alternate knee and hip.
Feel Agile and strong.
▽

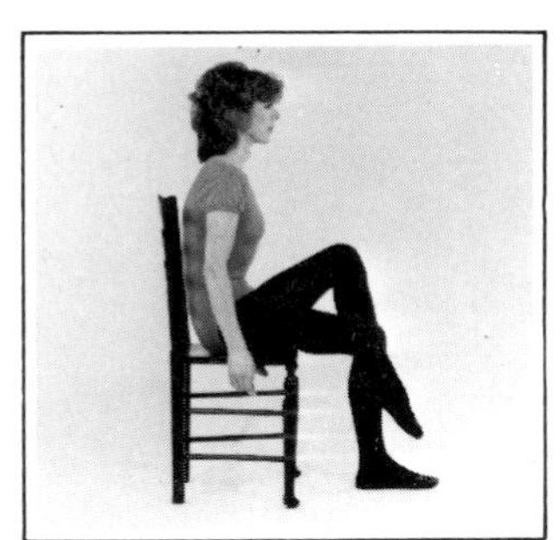

Good For Abdominals and back muscles.

THE SLIMNASTICS PROGRAMME

Week II
Healthy Eating Programme (less fat)

Begin by cutting down the fat in your diet.

- Buy low-fat spreads and use sparingly.
- Choose skimmed milk and limit your intake of cheese.
- Change your cooking methods (see 10 Steps p 20) and use recipes needing low-fat ingredients (see pp 25-40).
- Read the labels on any tins and watch any processed foods.

Remember that this step will benefit the health of everyone and for those who need to lose weight will cut dramatically their calorie intake.

Tension Control Technique (read and look)

This week after you have finished the 6 minutes of exercise, put on some warmer clothes and put your chair in front of a mirror and prop your book up where you can see it. Practise the TCT and watch yourself follow it. Note the tension in the body and its effects and also the results when you release the muscles completely. Again you can murmur the test out loud so that you can learn it. Allow yourself at least five minutes.

Weight this Week: .... st. .... lb.

The Slimnastics Exercises

Read the Safety Guidelines on p 18.

Wear comfortable clothing. Barefeet or non-slip shoes.

Week II Do each exercise for 1 minute.

Exercise One

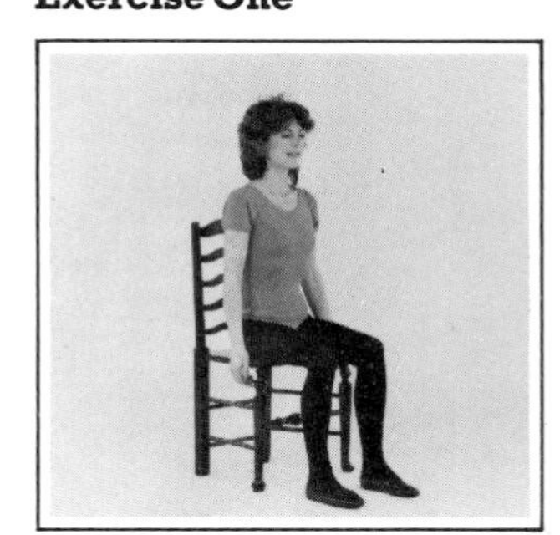

Start Sitting forward in chair, sit tall, feet apart on floor under knees. Arms by sides. Relax and breathe easily.

▽

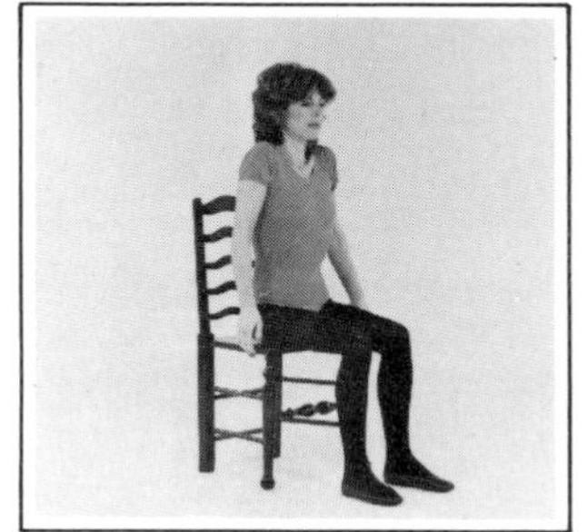

Exercise Circle shoulders, forwards, up, out and down.
Feel Exercise slow and spine stretched.

▽

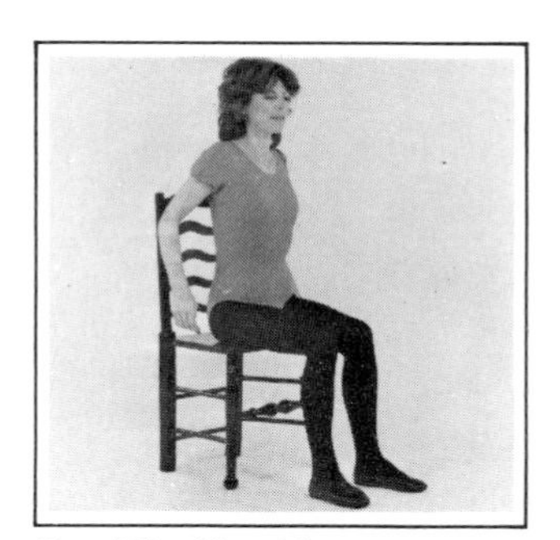

Good For Shoulders, arms, back. Relief of fatigue in shoulder area.

Exercise Two

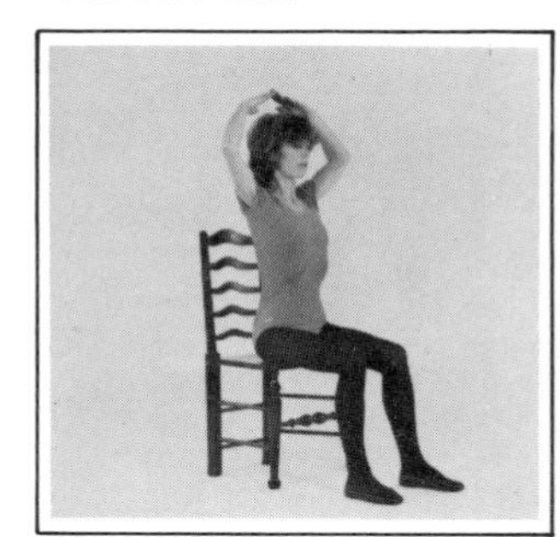

Start Sit tall, place hands lightly above head. Feet apart.

▽

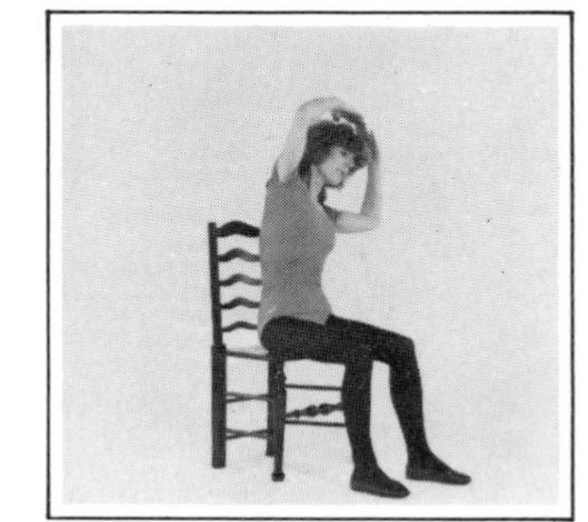

Exercise Bend over to one side then to the other side.
Feel Firm body and stretched rib cage.

▽

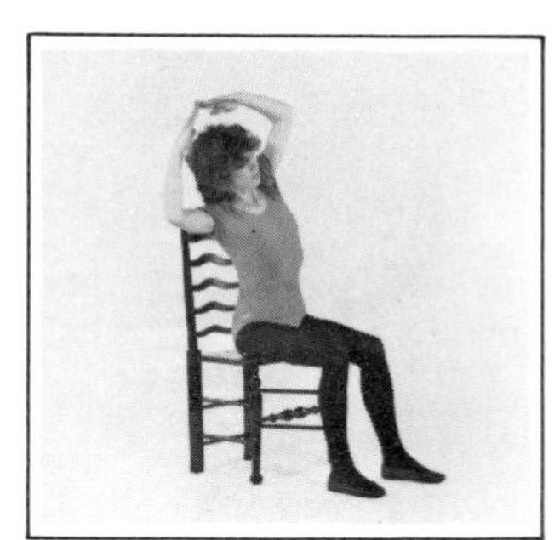

Good For Rib cage, spine and waist.

WEEK 2

Exercise Three

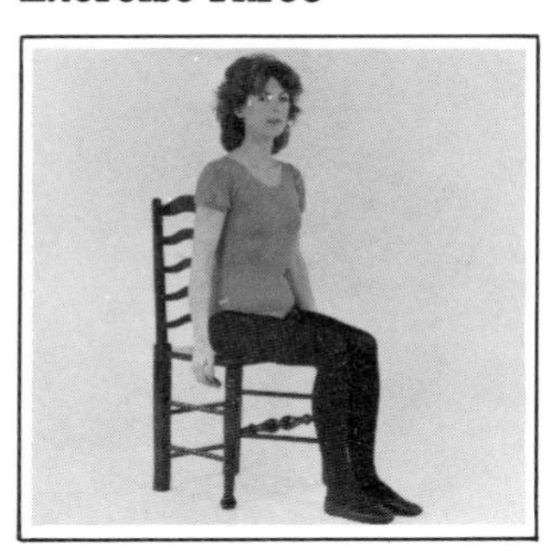

Start Sit tall.

▽

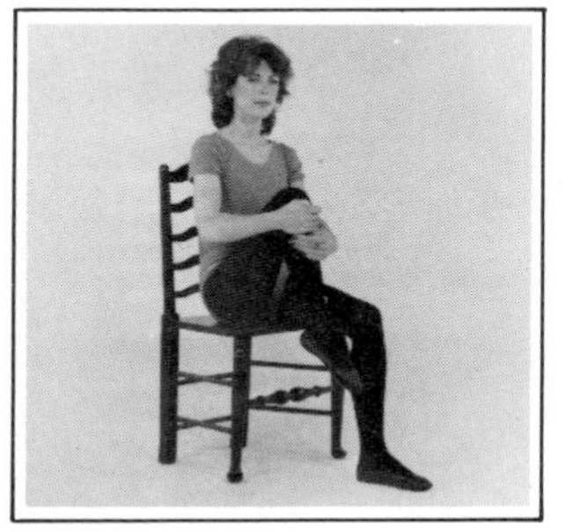

Exercise Bend one leg and pull gently to chest.
Feel Back straight and body balanced.

▽

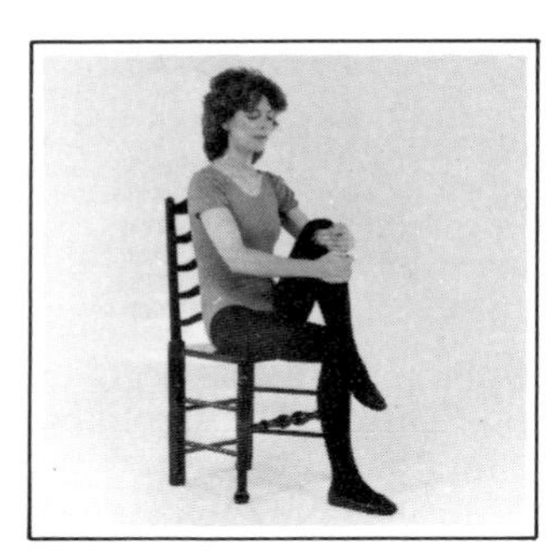

Good For Hip and knee mobility.

Exercise Four

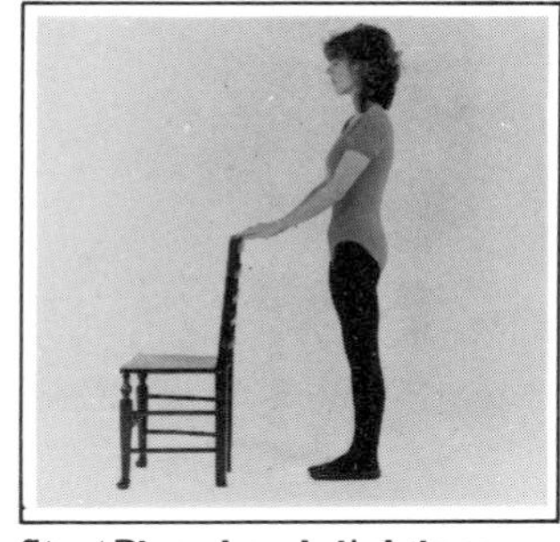

Start Place hands lightly on chair back. Stand tall, feet together and parallel. Relax shoulders, breathe easily.

▽

Exercise Bend knees forwards, keep heels on floor, then go up on tip toes.
Feel Tall and strong.

▽

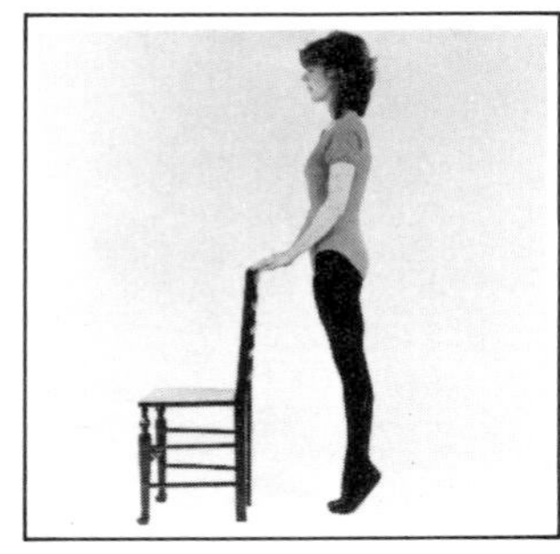

Good For Posture, legs and thighs.

Exercise Five

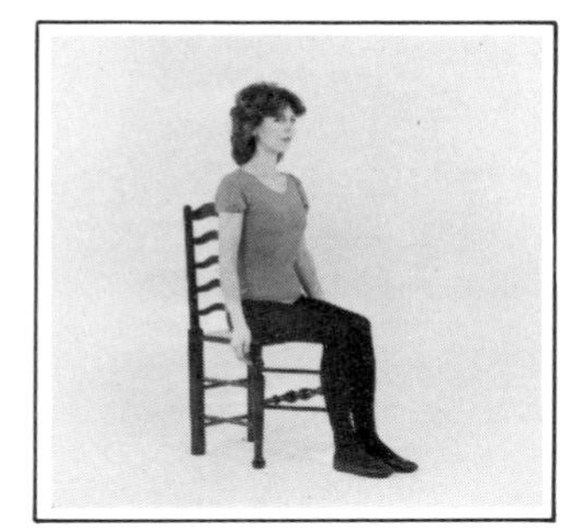

Start Sit tall.

▽

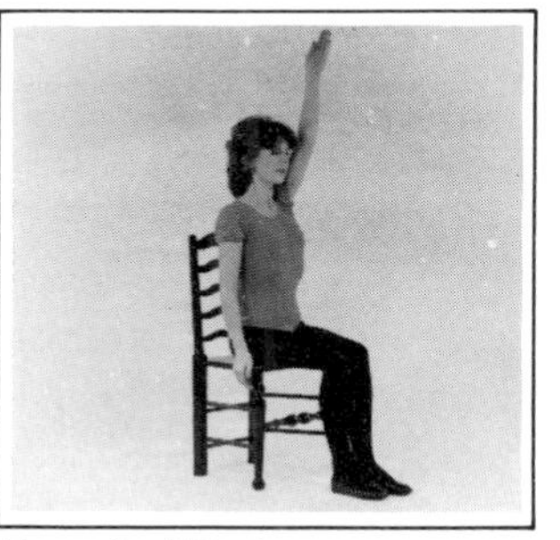

Exercise Lift alternate arms above head.
Feel Slow exercise, stretched firm spine.

▽

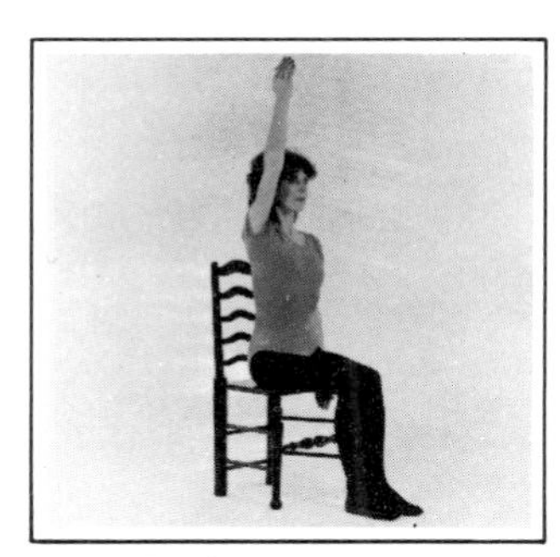

Good For Shoulder mobility and back strength.

Exercise Six

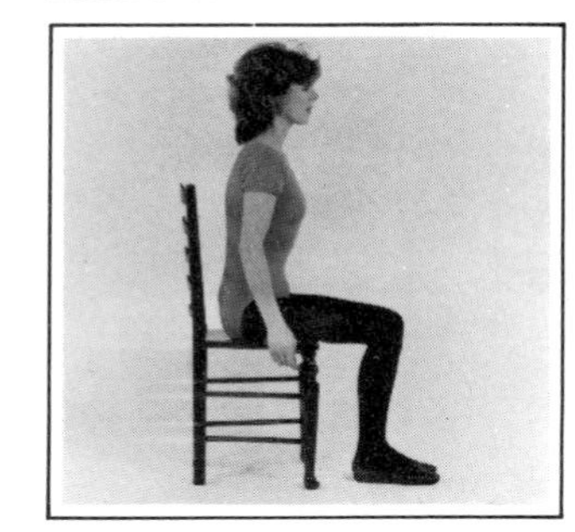

Start Sit tall.

▽

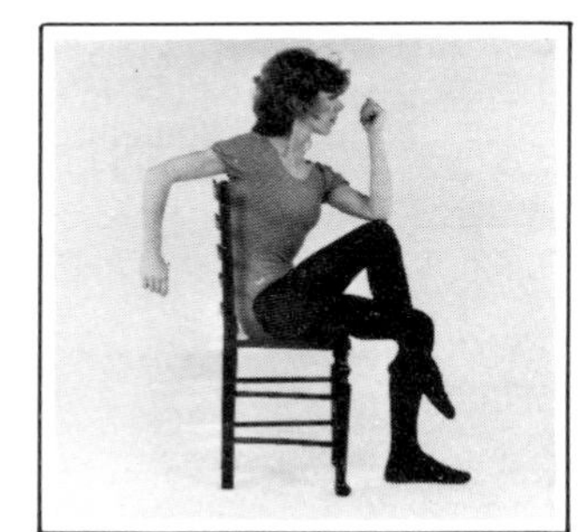

Exercise Lift knee to reach opposite elbow. Turn trunk.
Feel Continuous exercise, strong and agile spine.

▽

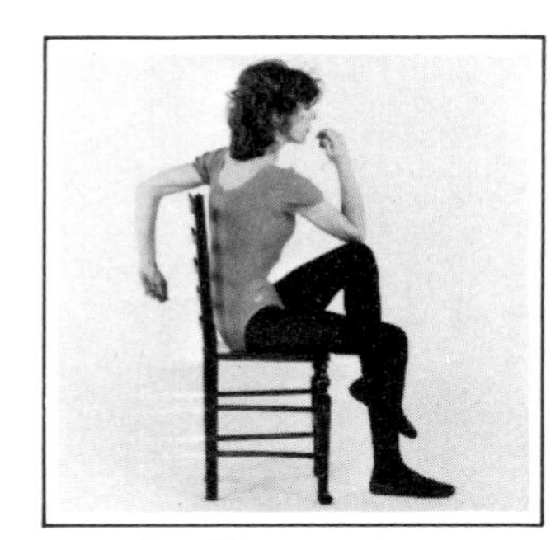

Good For Waist, back and spine.

THE SLIMNASTICS PROGRAMME

Week III

Healthy Eating Programme (cereals)

The next step is to introduce some more cereals into your meals.

- Make wholemeal bread from recipe on p 25.
- Cereals or extra fibre for breakfast are essential – why not try porridge?
- Look at the shopping list for more cereal foods and bring some of them into your menu for the week. Remember brown rice and wholemeal pasta.
- Potatoes can come in here too. Forget their 'old' image and include them (with their skins and without any extra fat).

You do not need to be hungry or empty when you are eating healthily!

Tension Control Technique (memorising)

By now you will be ready to do the technique without the aid of written notes. After the exercise session put on warm clothes and this time lie on the bed or if you have had back trouble of any kind, lie on a sleeping bag or covering on the floor with perhaps a pillow under your head. If you find it difficult to lie down, sit in a chair (making sure your head, neck and body are supported). Close your eyes and carefully follow the routine. Again if it makes it easier murmur the text out loud and in any event say it deliberately and slowly, following the directions, holding and completely releasing each time.

Weight this Week .... st. .... lb.

The Slimnastics Exercises

Read the Safety Guidelines on p 18.

Wear comfortable clothing. Barefeet or non-slip shoes.

Week III Do each exercise for 1 minute.

Exercise One

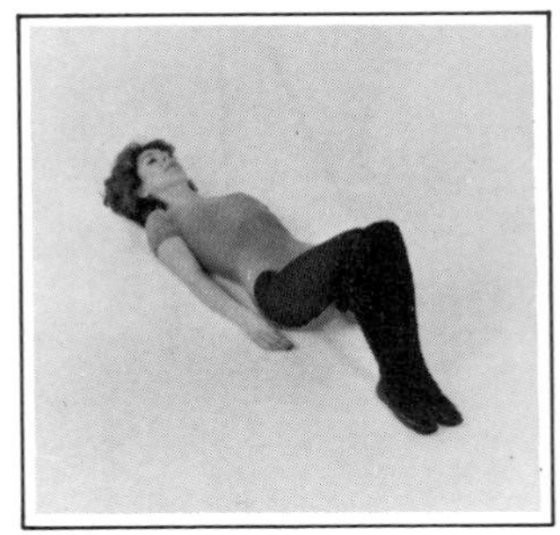

Start Crook lying, press back into floor, long neck, stretch spine, keep breathing regularly.

▽

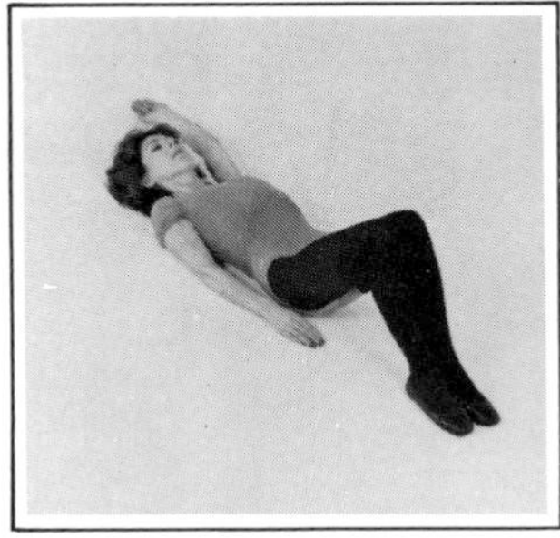

Exercise Lift alternate arms above head as far as you can.
Feel Tummy and back firm – exercise slow.

▽

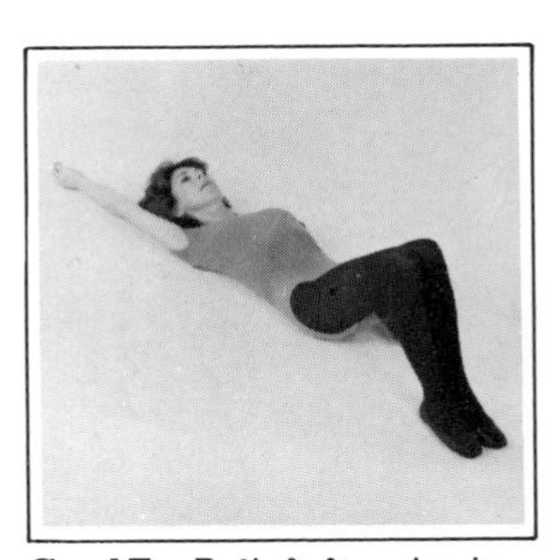

Good For Relief of tension in shoulders. Loosens shoulder girdle and joints.

Exercise Two

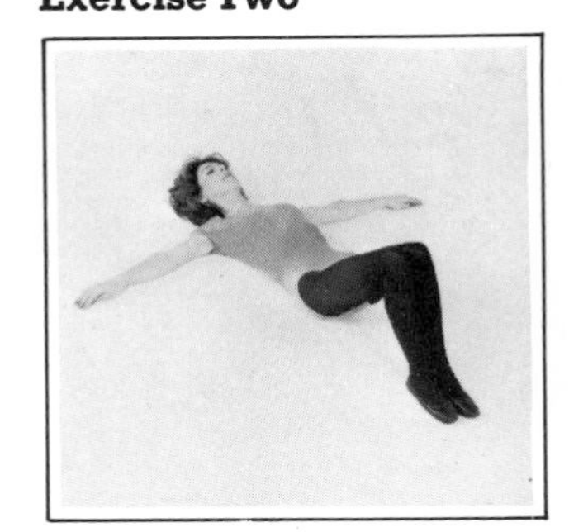

Start Arms sideways, keep shoulders and feet on floor.

▽

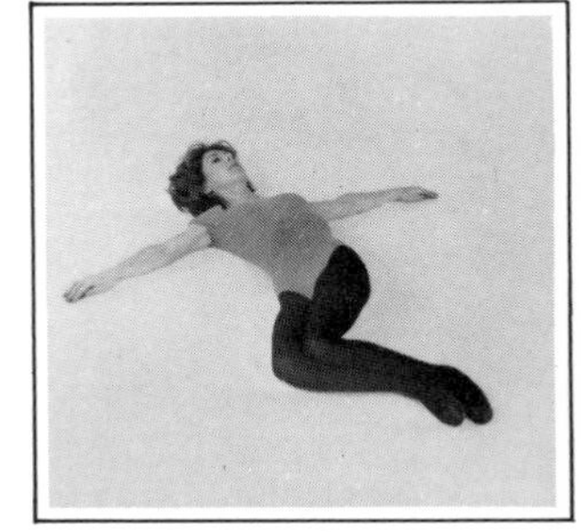

Exercise Lower knees to alternate sides.
Feel Spine twisted and exercise controlled.

▽

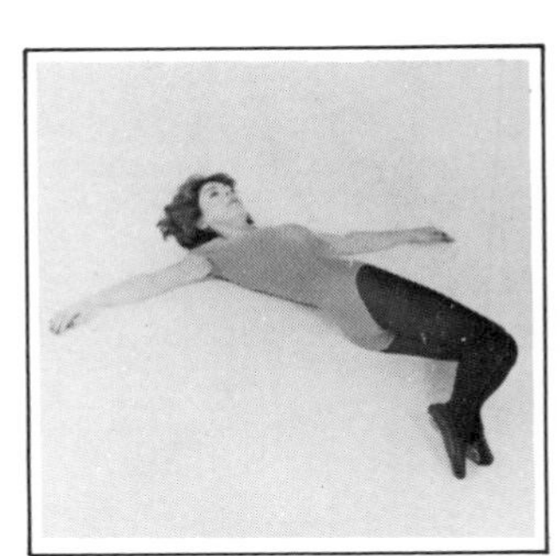

Good For Waist line and spine mobility.

WEEK 3

Exercise Three

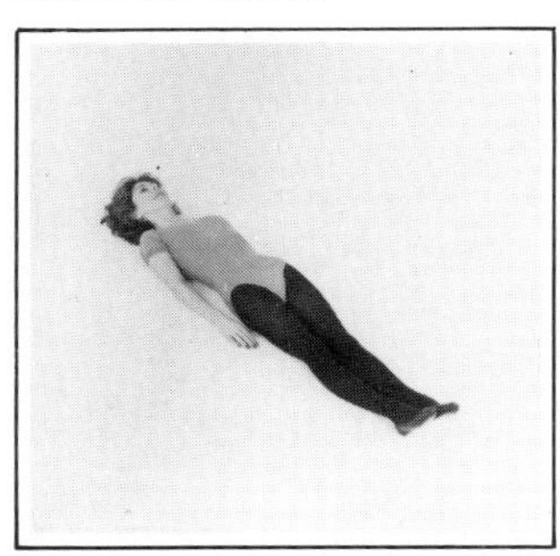

Start Lying. Press back into floor – stretch spine.

▽

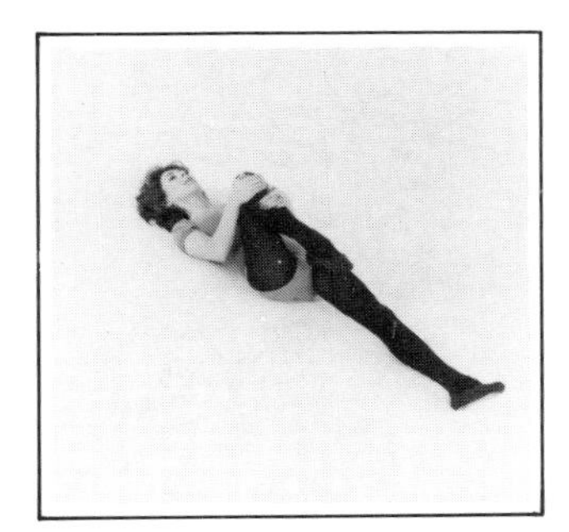

Exercise Bend one leg, hold it and circle the ankle, repeat with other leg.
Feel Tummy firm and joints stretched.

▽

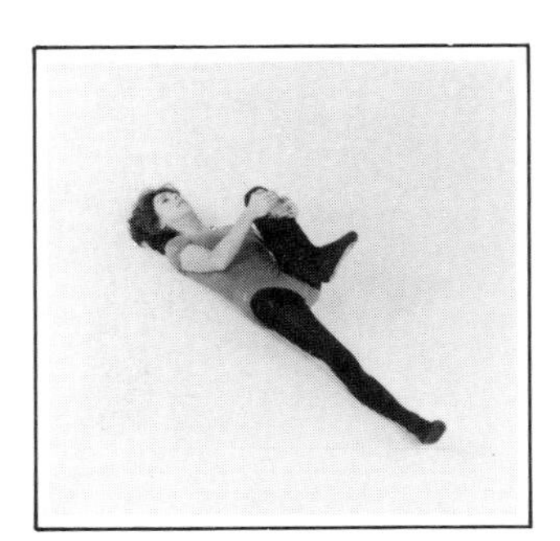

Good For Mobility of hip, knee and ankle.

Exercise Four

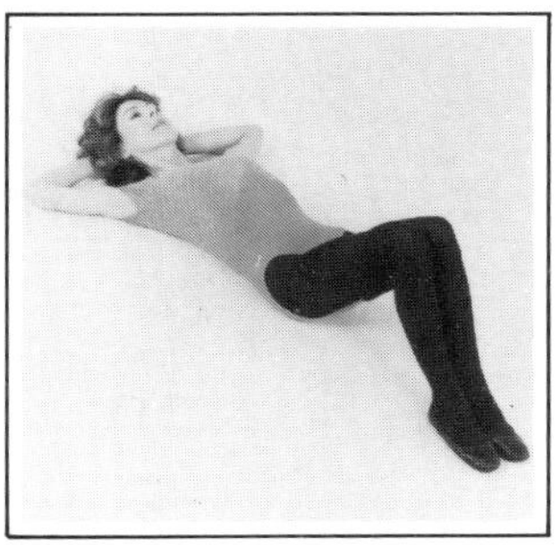

Start Crook lying, hands behind head, elbows sideways. Press back into floor.

▽

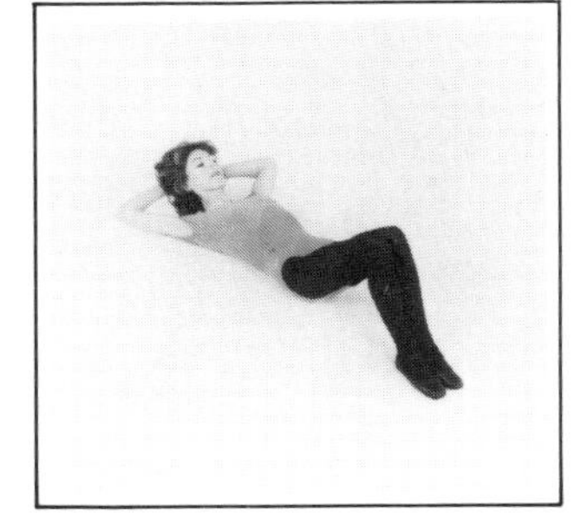

Exercise Slowly lift head and lower. Support head lightly only.
Feel Tummy strong and easy, continuous movement.

▽

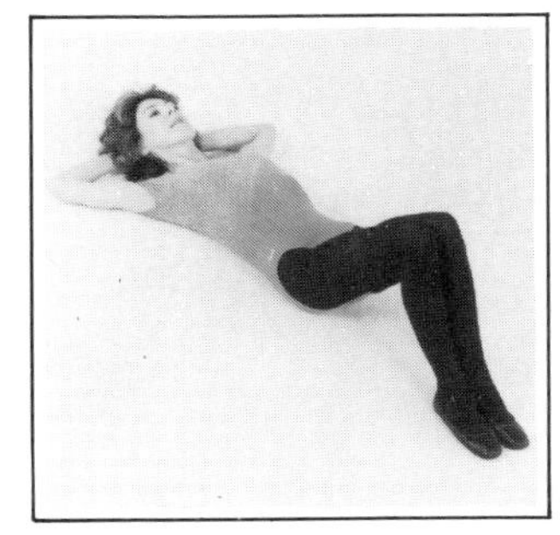

Good For Neck, abdominal muscles and shoulders.

Exercise Five

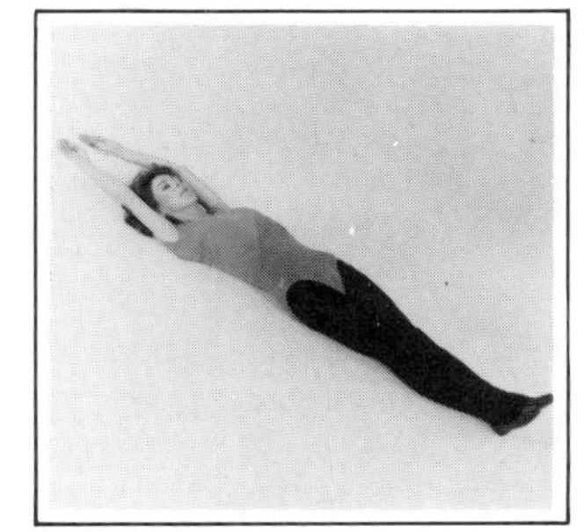

Start Lying with stretched arms, spine and legs.

▽

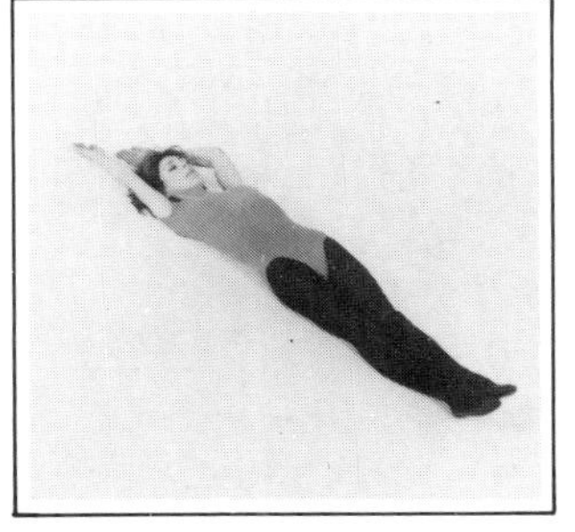

Exercise Make one arm longer than the other. Then make one leg longer than the other – slowly.
Feel Stretched and relaxed.

▽

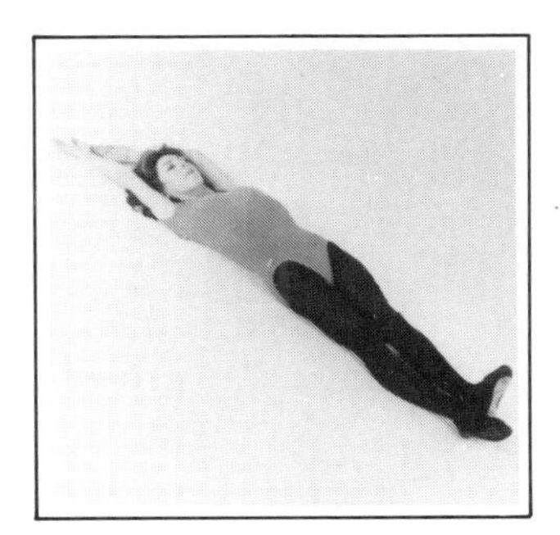

Good For Relief of tension. Stretched spine arms and legs.

Exercise Six

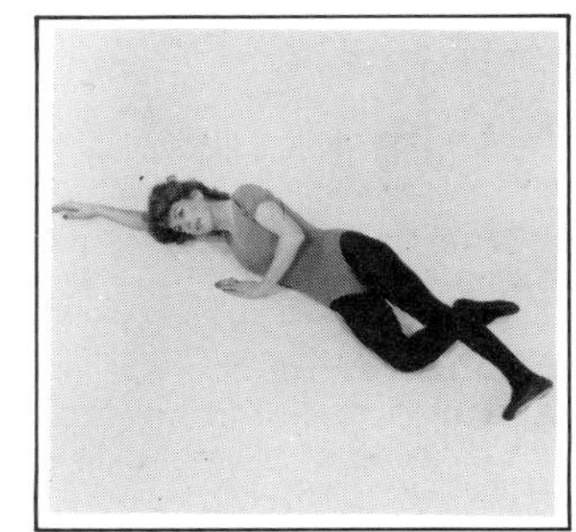

Start Side lying, top leg straight with foot flexed, knee facing forwards.

▽

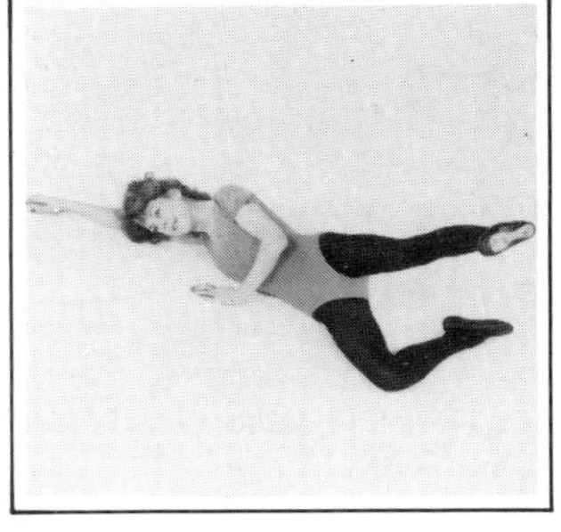

Exercise Lift leg straight up and down keeping foot parallel to floor. Keep knee and foot facing forwards.
Feel Strong movement and balanced body.

▽

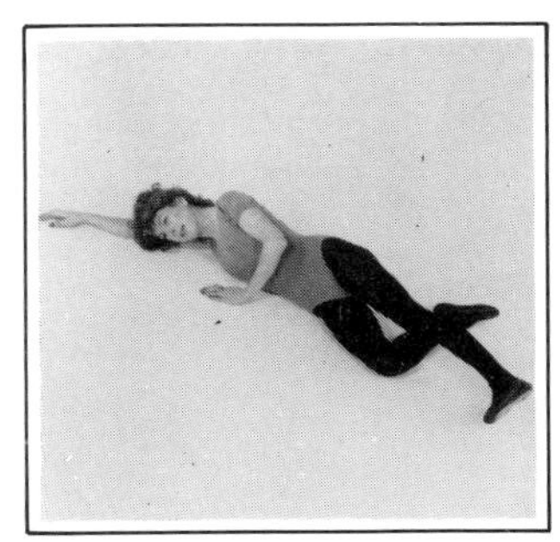

Good For Outer thighs and hips.

THE SLIMNASTICS PROGRAMME

Week IV
Healthy Eating Programme (no refined carbohydrates)

This week, continuing to remember to cut down the fats and have some cereals, cut out the unnecessary foods from your meals. This means those containing sugar and refined flours. There is a long list of these under No.3 in the 10 Steps on p 20.

Favourites though some of these foods are, sugar adds nothing nutritional to our diet except calories and it is thought to actively do us some harm as well. Also remember that foods containing sugar (such as dried fruits) are equally fattening.

Tension Control Technique (reactions to stress)

Continue to practise the relaxation every day after the exercise session. Start being aware when you feel or react to tension during your working day or home life. If you notice the tension or feel the physical results such as 'butterflies in your stomach' or the others noted on p 40 make a conscious effort to tighten up your muscles quite deliberately and forcefully. Then let them release. Do this several times and you will find yourself calming down.

Weight this Week .... st. .... lb.

The Slimnastics Exercises

Read the Safety Guidelines on p 18.

Wear comfortable clothing. Barefeet or non-slip shoes.

Week IV Do exercises for 1 minute each.

Exercise One

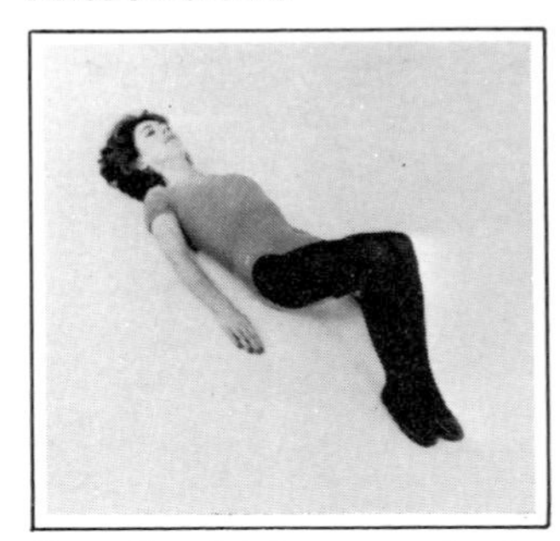

Start Crook lying, press back into floor, long neck, stretch spine, keep breathing regularly.
▽

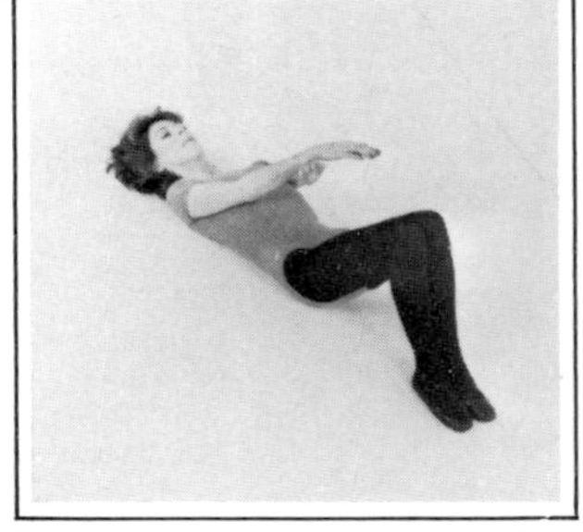

Exercise Cross arms over chest and place out sideways on floor.
Feel Stretched arms and shoulders and a firm spine.
▽

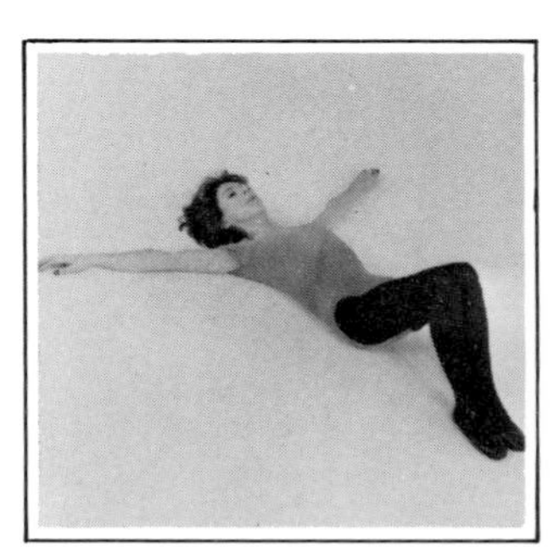

Good For Arms and thorax, breathing.

Exercise Two

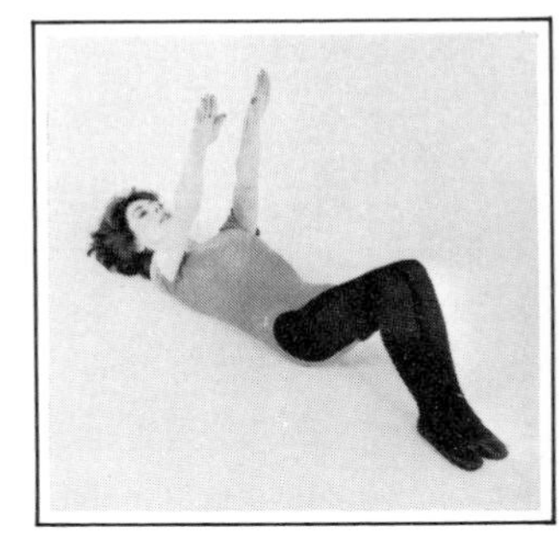

Start Crook lying, knees and feet still.
▽

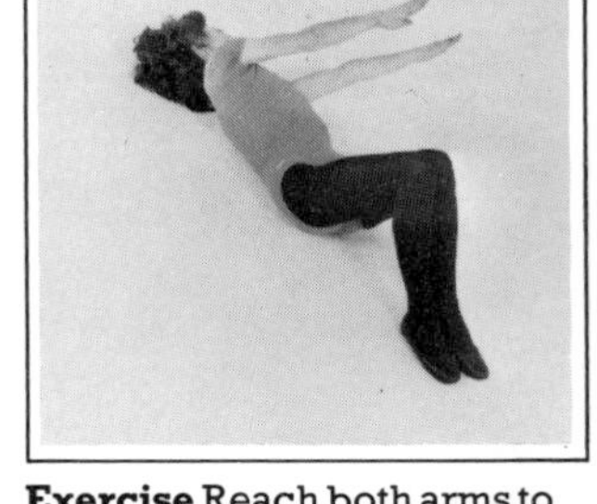

Exercise Reach both arms to ceiling and lower on alternate sides. Turn head and trunk with arms.
Feel Twisted spine and stretched arms and shoulders.
▽

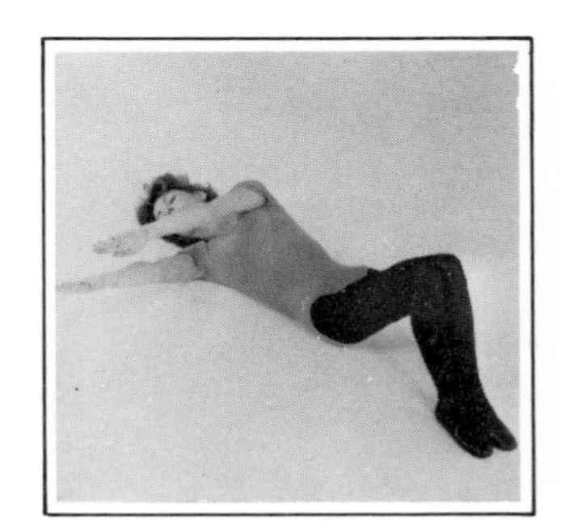

Good For Upper spine, neck and arms.

WEEK 4

Exercise Three

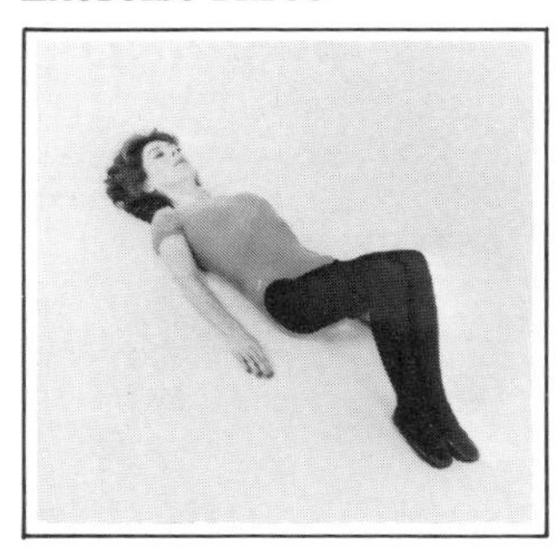

Start Crook lying. Stretch spine and firm buttocks.
▽

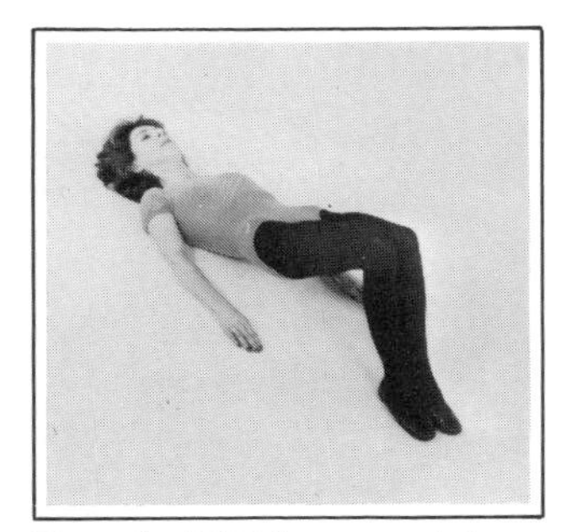

Exercise Lift hips up and down. Do not lift rib cage or arch the spine.
Feel Straight spine and small, slow movement.
▽

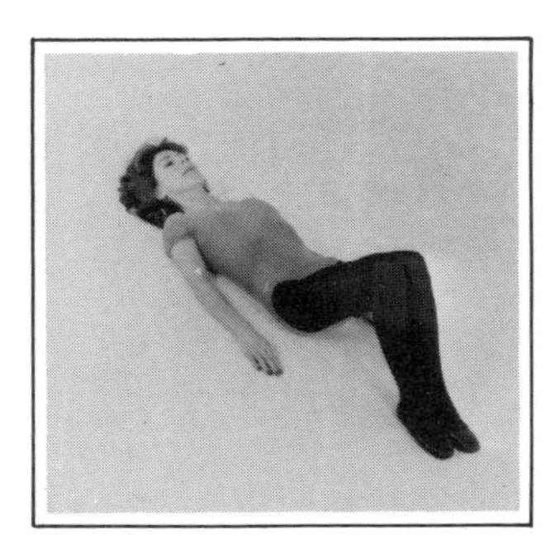

Good For Back and pelvic floor and buttocks.

Exercise Four

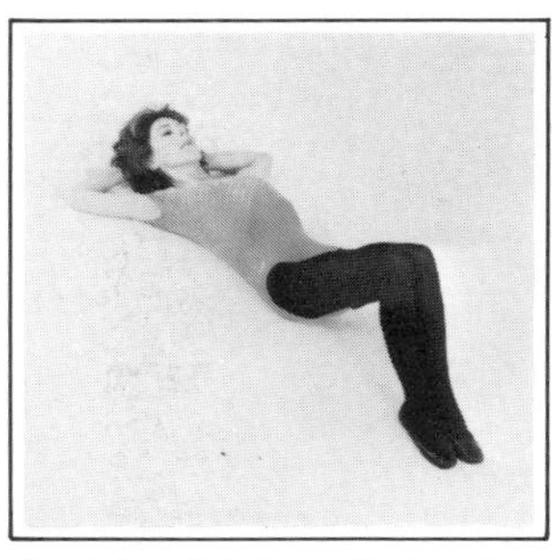

Start Crook lying with hands lightly under head, elbows out sideways. Press back into floor.
▽

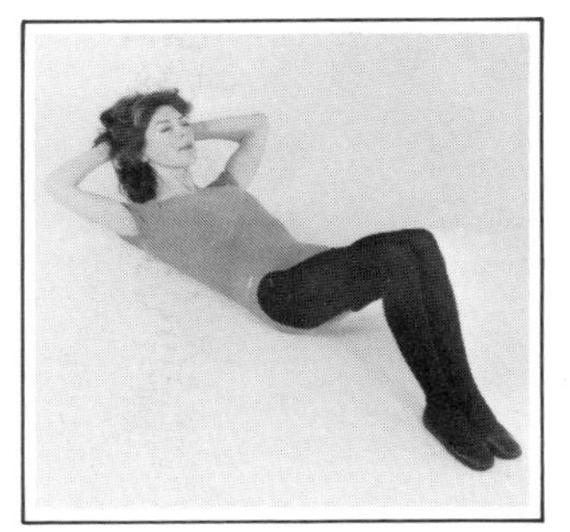

Exercise Lift head, shoulders and arms off floor and shorten tummy muscles. Keep breathing regularly. Hold elbows back and look towards the ceiling.
Feel Strong and rhythmical.
▽

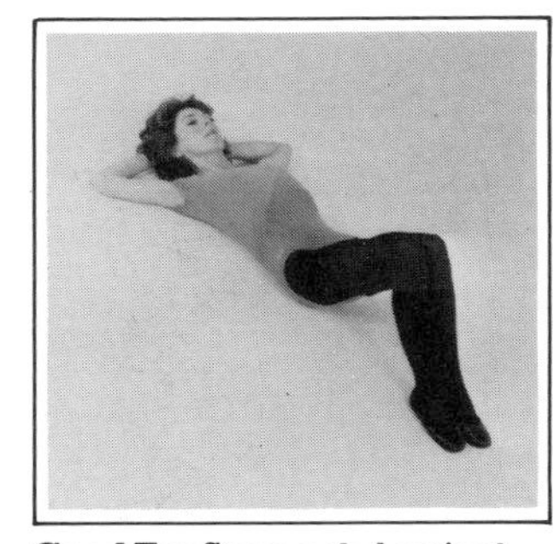

Good For Strong abdominal muscles.

Exercise Five

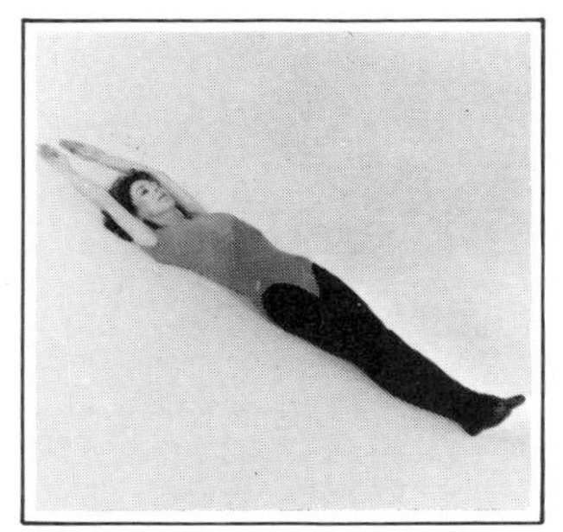

Start Stretched lying – keep breathing – press back into floor.
▽

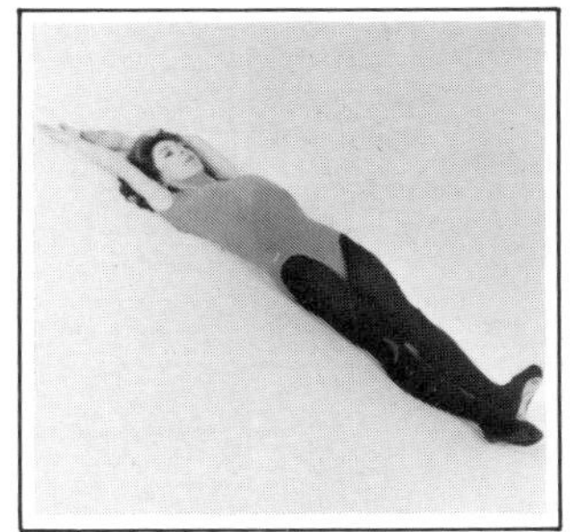

Exercise Make one leg and same arm as long as possible – then the other.
Feel Arms and legs stretched and slow reaching movement.
▽

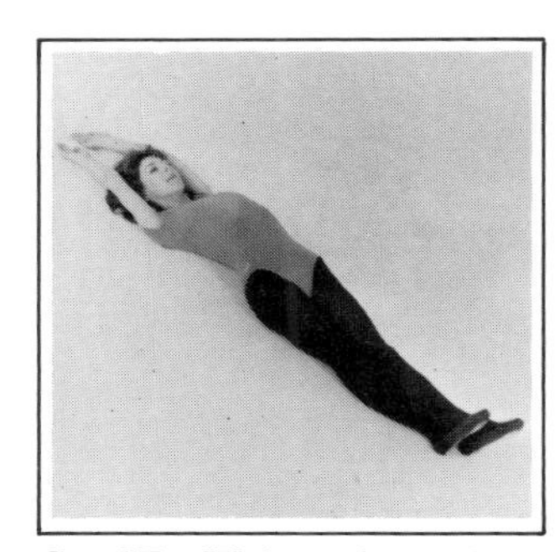

Good For Waist, spine and relief of tension.

Exercise Six

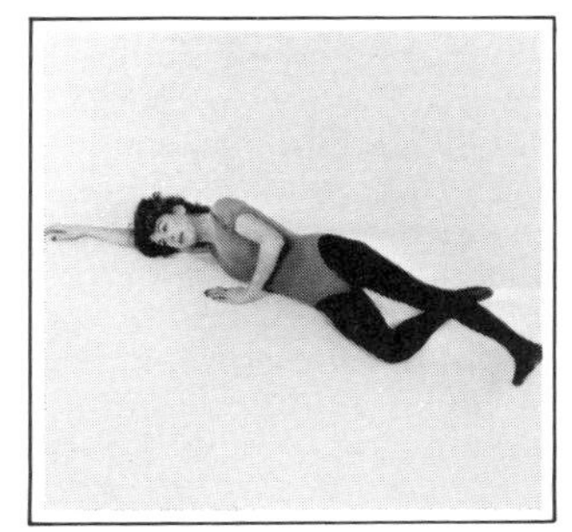

Start Side lying – top leg straight, foot flexed, knee facing forwards.
▽

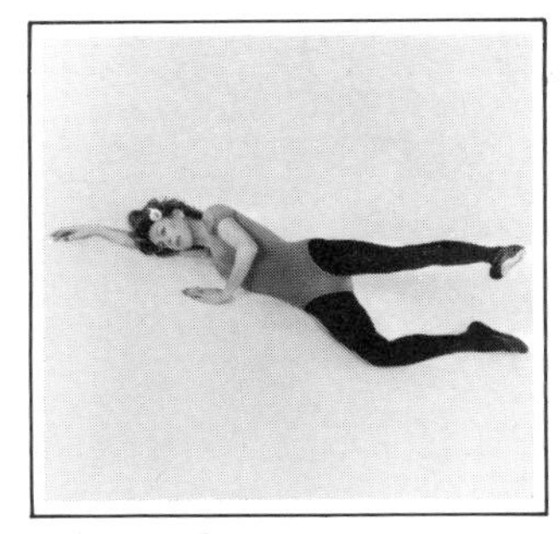

Exercise Circle top leg keeping straight.
Feel Body balanced and firm, strong movement.
▽

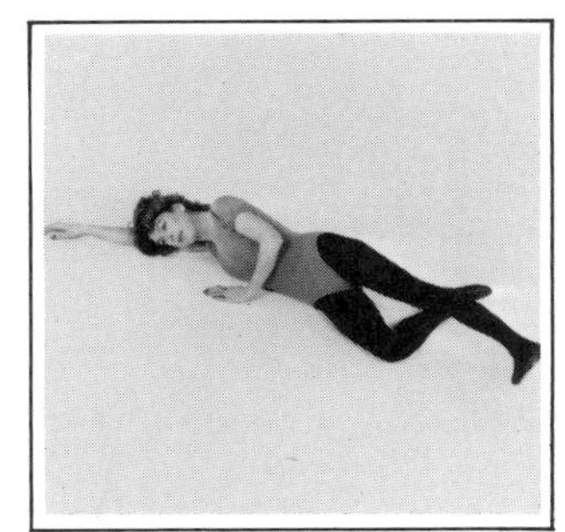

Good For Firm buttocks, bottom and thighs and circulation.

THE SLIMNASTICS PROGRAMME

Week V

Healthy Eating Programme (vegetables)

Now is the time to start being more adventurous! Look round your supermarket or greengrocer for some unfamiliar or neglected (by you) vegetables and buy them and try them this week.

Look at our recipes and read the shopping lists. Vegetables as well as being an excellent source of fibre are full of vitamins and other nutrients which help to keep us healthy (see the charts in the appendix).

They have exciting tastes and many lovely colours. Eat as many as you can in salads too.

Tension Control Technique (tension in life)

Continue to practise the TCT every day after the 6 minutes of exercises. Also continue becoming aware of tension during your everyday life. Now deliberately pre-empt 'stress moments' and start to tighten and release, tighten and release (privately and discreetly) when you are aware that a situation is about to or might arise. You will find that you will be able to cope with a clearer more able mind and will not suffer the results of 'over tension' afterwards.

Weight this Week: .... st. .... lb.

The Slimnastics Exercises

Read the Safety Guidelines on p 18.

Wear comfortable clothing. Barefeet or non-slip shoes.

Week V Do each exercise for 1 minute.

Exercise One

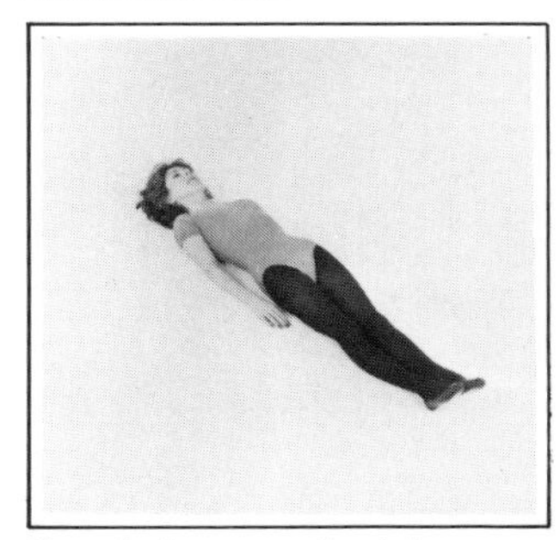

Start Lying stretched, long spine and neck, relaxed arms and fingers.

▽

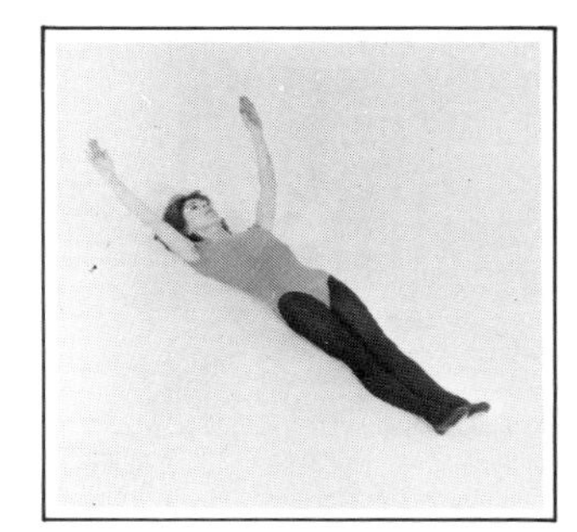

Exercise Lift arms over and above head sideways and back to start. Press back into the floor. Keep breathing naturally.
Feel A firm body, easy arm movements.

▽

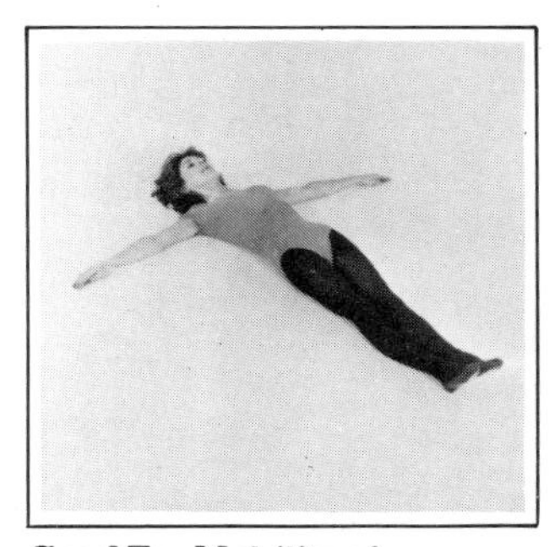

Good For Mobility of shoulders, relaxation and stretch.

Exercise Two

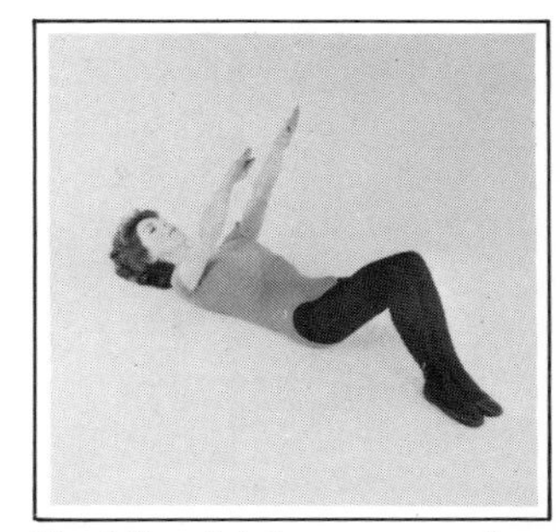

Start Crook lying, press spine into floor, firm stomach and buttocks.

▽

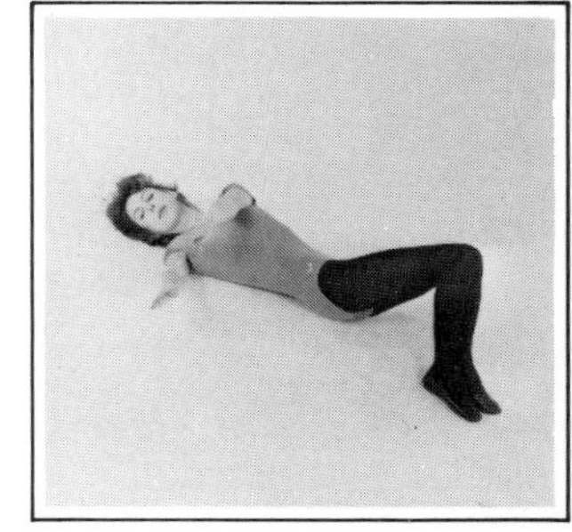

Exercise Lower both knees to one side and both arms to other side at the same time. Repeat other side. Head follows the arms.
Feel Slow stretched movement and rotated spine.

▽

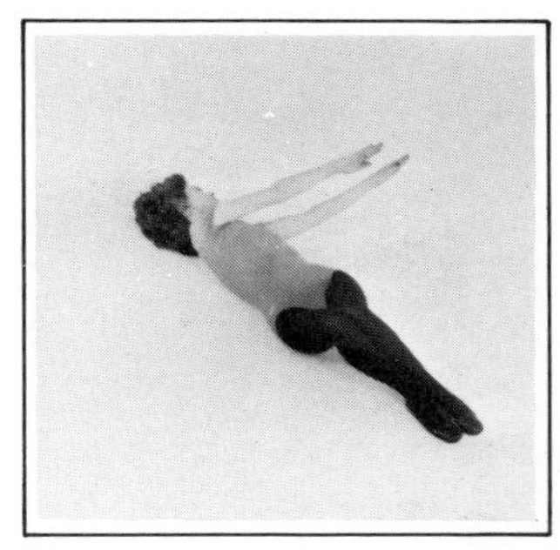

Good For Spine and waist, arms and shoulders.

WEEK 5

Exercise Three

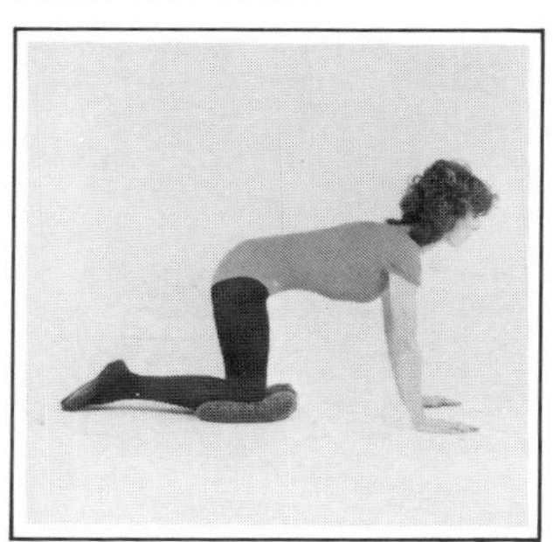

Start Prone kneeling. Hands under shoulders, knees under hips. Straight spine.
▽

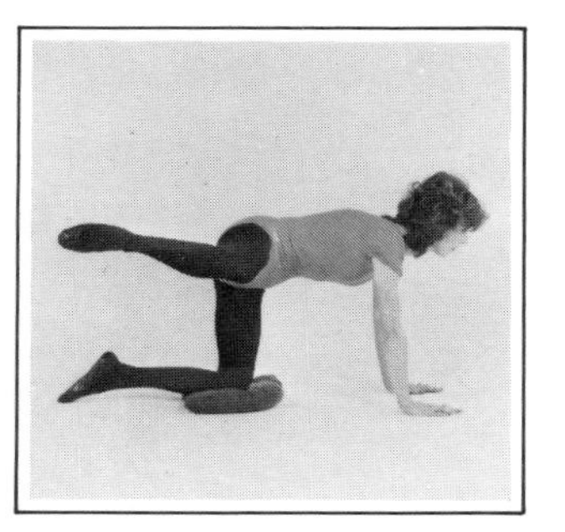

Exercise Lift thigh and bend leg sideways continuously.
Feel Balanced, slow and strong leg lift.
▽

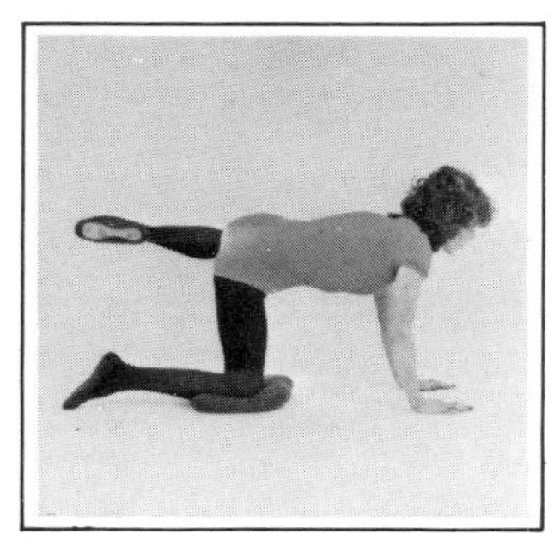

Good For Thighs and buttocks.

Exercise Four

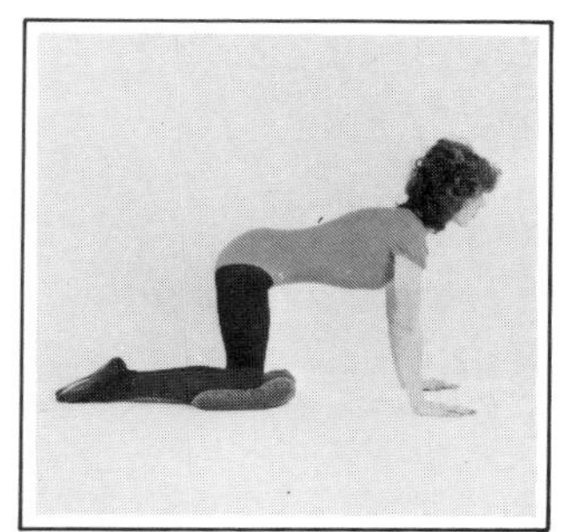

Start Prone kneeling.
▽

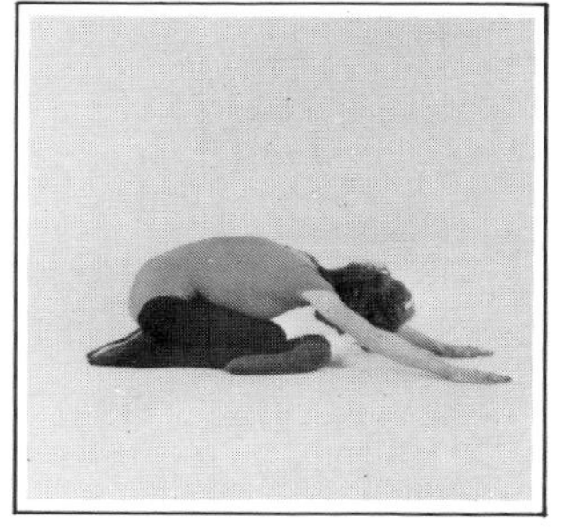

Exercise Slowly go backwards with hips and lower hips towards heels.
Feel Strong body and stretched joints.
▽

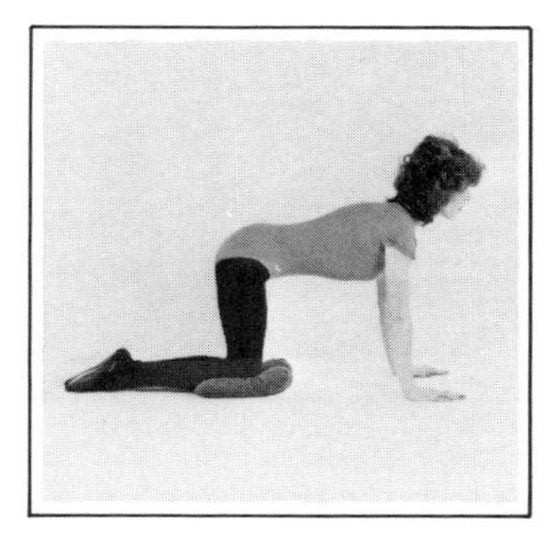

Good For Shoulder stretch. Hip and knee mobility. Back muscles.

Exercise Five

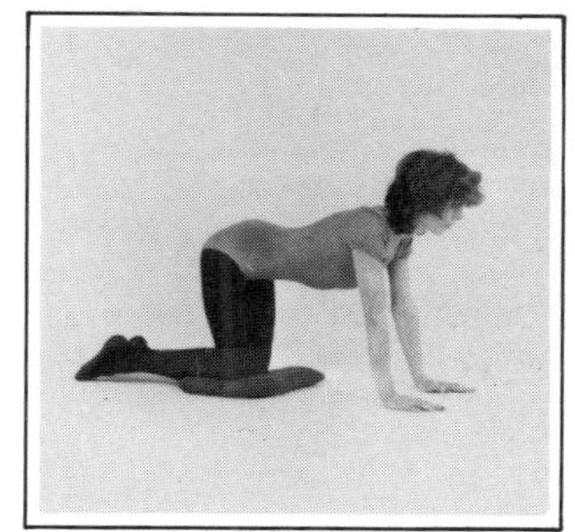

Start Prone kneeling.
▽

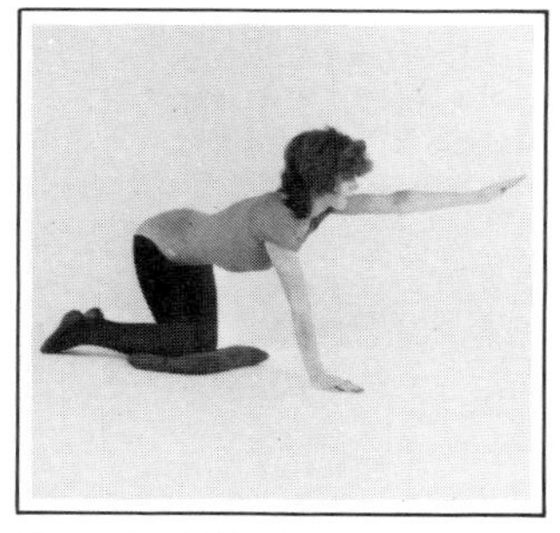

Exercise Lift alternate arms, then lift alternate legs.
Feel Stretched, strong and long.
▽

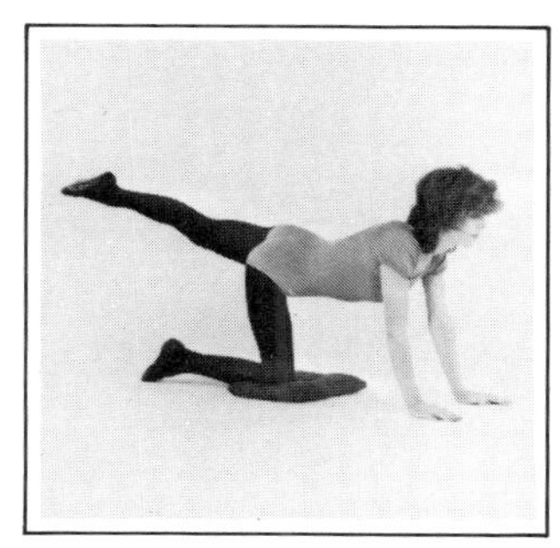

Good For Back and buttocks.

Exercise Six

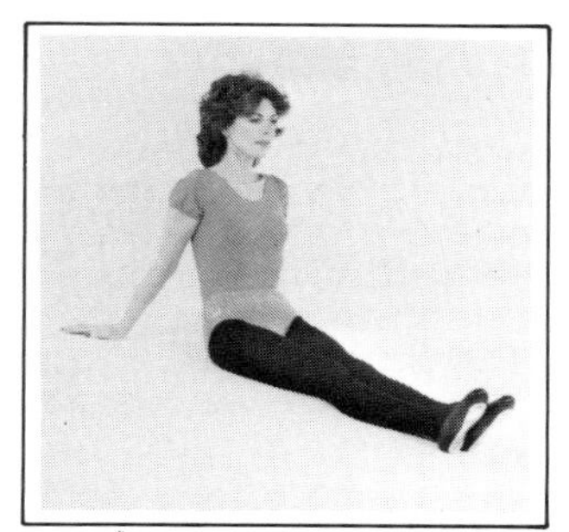

Start Sitting, relaxed knees, legs straight, strong back.
▽

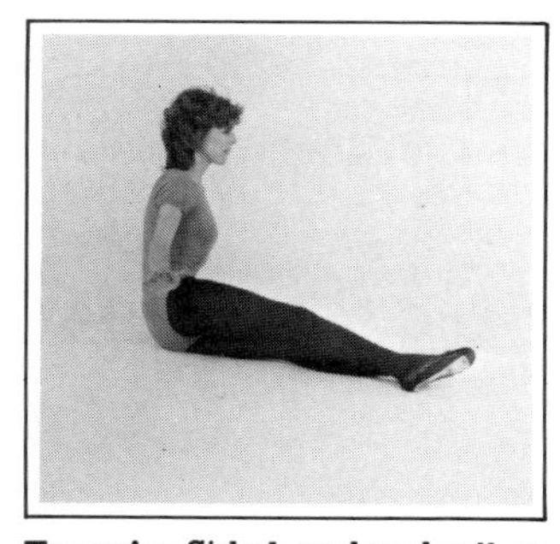

Exercise Side bend and roll on to alternate buttock.
Feel Slow and rhythmical.
▽

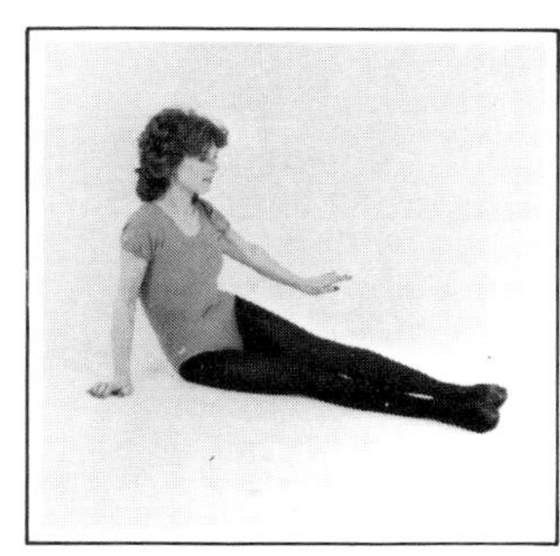

Good For Waist and buttocks.

THE SLIMNASTICS PROGRAMME

Week VI
Healthy Eating Programme (pulses)

This week include more pulses. They are often a much neglected part of our possible foods and yet they have so much to offer as they contain protein as well as fibre and other nutrients. They can play an important part in our effort to cut down on animal protein so this week use them to stretch small portions of meat, or even in dishes of their own.

Look at our shopping lists in the appendix and read the recipes on p 28.

There are many books available with recipes and ideas. Magazines are full of them too.

Tension Control Technique (work off steam)

Continue to practise the TCT both after the exercise session and at any time you need it.

This week take steps to find a good way to work off steam if you ever get truly 'uptight'. It might be that a metal dustbin and a collection of broken crockery kept together available for noisy throwing (a bottle bank is an even better and more constructive way of making a crashing din!) or kneading that wholemeal bread, or dancing to music or perhaps walking the dog is the way that suits you best. It is good to discover your safety valve and remember to use it rather than let the tension do you harm.

Weight this Week .... st. .... lb.

The Slimnastics Exercises

Read the Safety Guidelines on p 18.

Wear comfortable clothing. Barefeet or non-slip shoes.

Week VI Do each exercise for 1 minute.

Exercise One

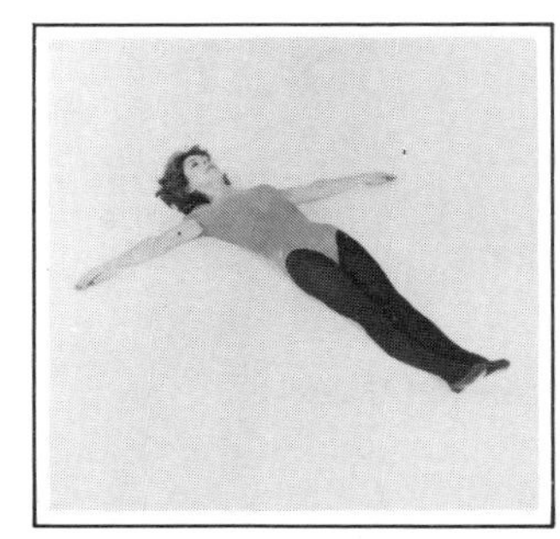

Start Lying stretched, spine and neck long, relaxed arms and fingers.
▽

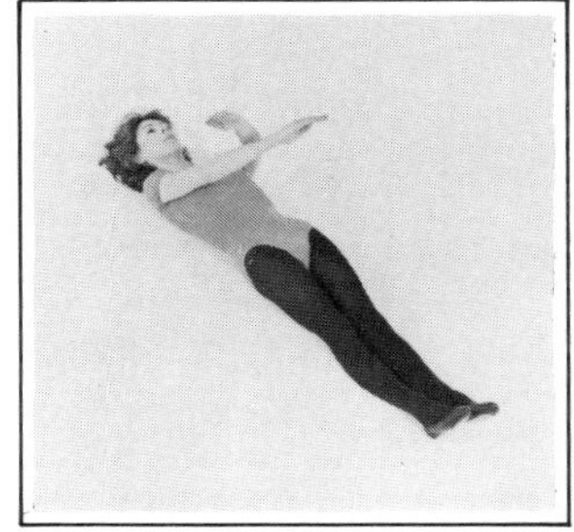

Exercise Arms circling and going in opposite directions over body and above head.
Feel Stretched arms and firm back.
▽

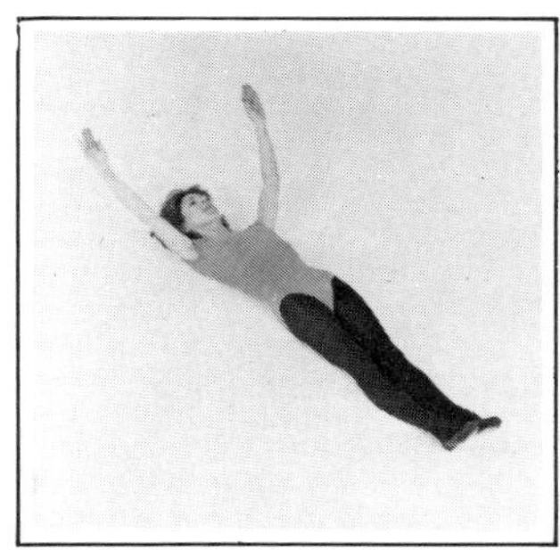

Good For Circulation and mobility in shoulders and arms.

Exercise Two

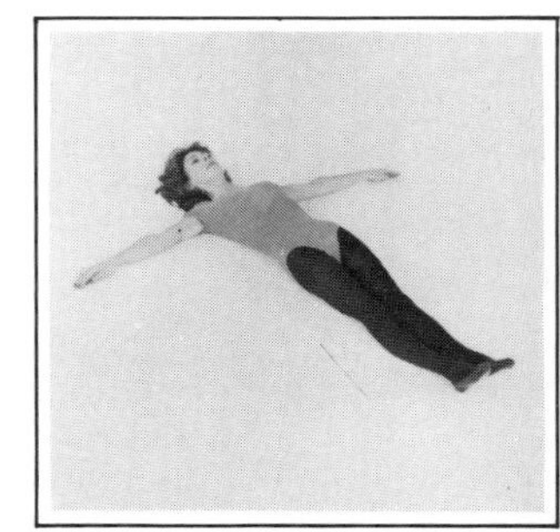

Start Lying, press spine into floor, firm stomach and buttocks. Arms out sideways, legs straight.
▽

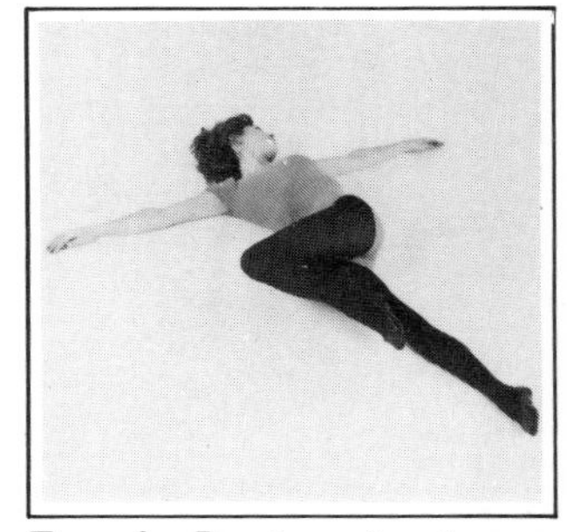

Exercise Bend one leg, lower knee towards floor, crossing over straight leg. Keep shoulders and arms still. Turn head opposite way to bent leg.
Feel Strong, slow movement, rotated spine.
▽

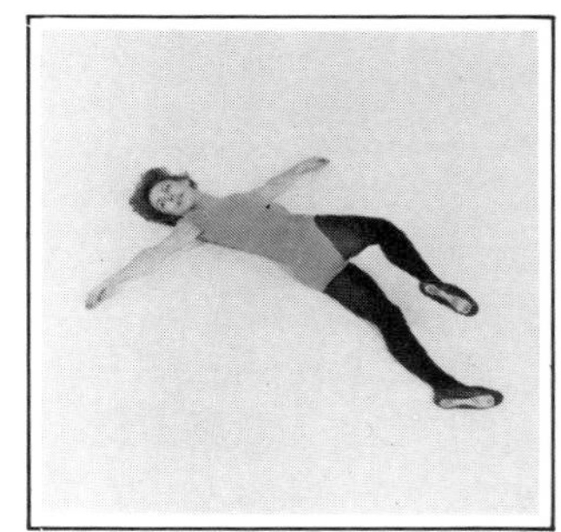

Good For Spine and back mobility and strengthening abdominals.

WEEK 6

Exercise Three

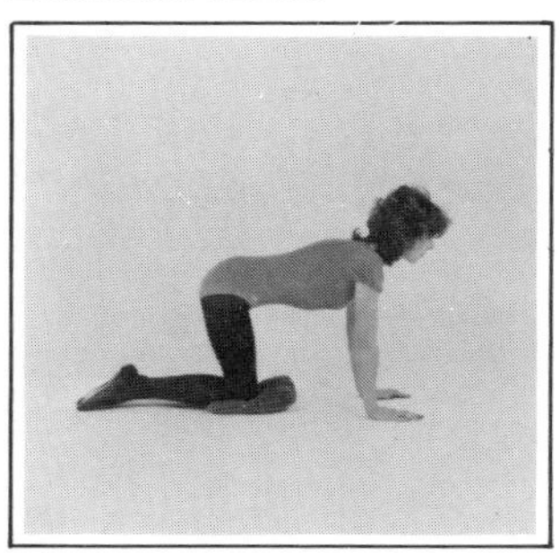

Start Prone kneeling, hands under shoulders, knees under hips.
▽

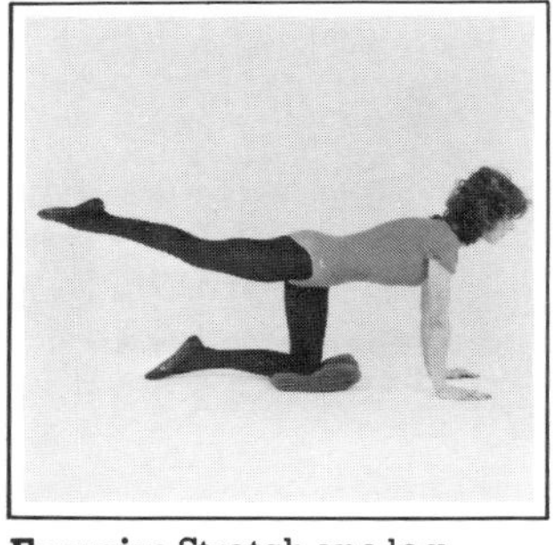

Exercise Stretch one leg behind. Keeping leg straight move out to side and behind again.
Feel Balanced body, slow and swinging movement.
▽

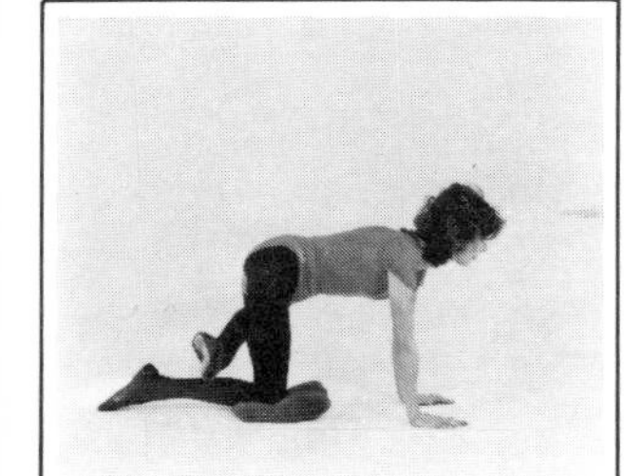

Good For Buttocks, lower back and thighs.

Exercise Four

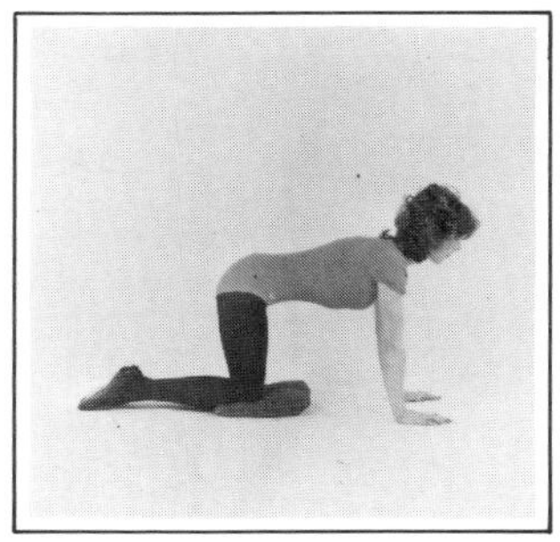

Start Prone kneeling.
▽

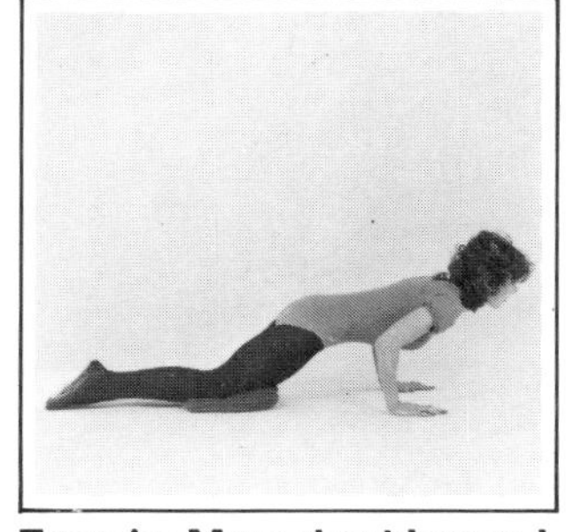

Exercise Move shoulders and body forwards to lying. Keep back and tummy straight.
Feel Slow, strong movement.
▽

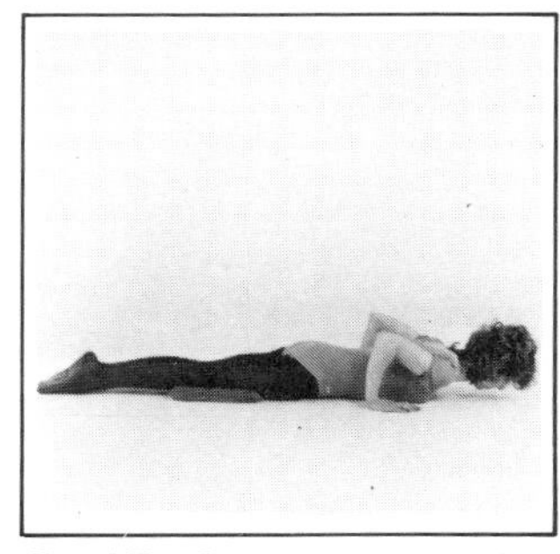

Good For Posture, arms and stomach muscles.

Exercise Five

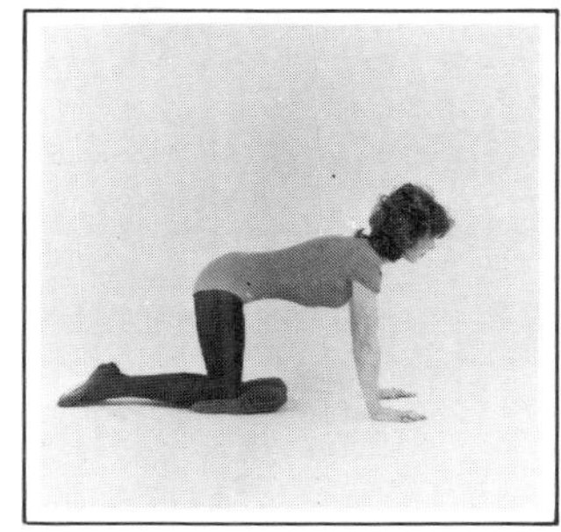

Start Prone kneeling.
▽

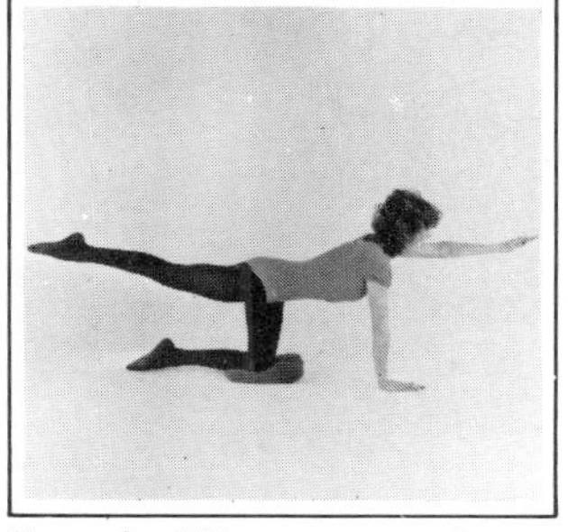

Exercise Lift one arm and opposite leg at same time. Repeat other side.
Feel Stretched, strong and long.
▽

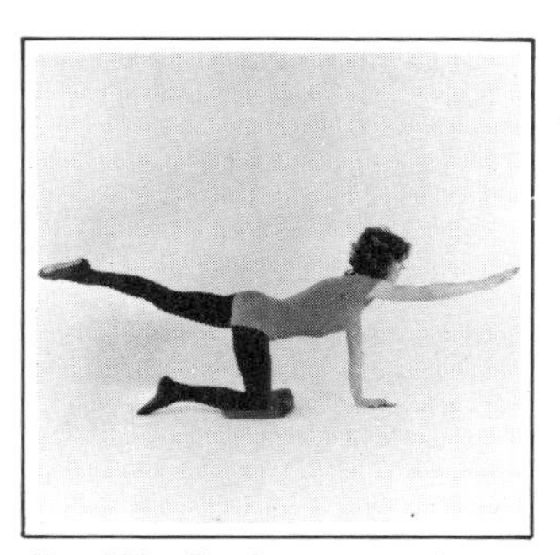

Good For Back, arms and legs and balance.

Exercise Six

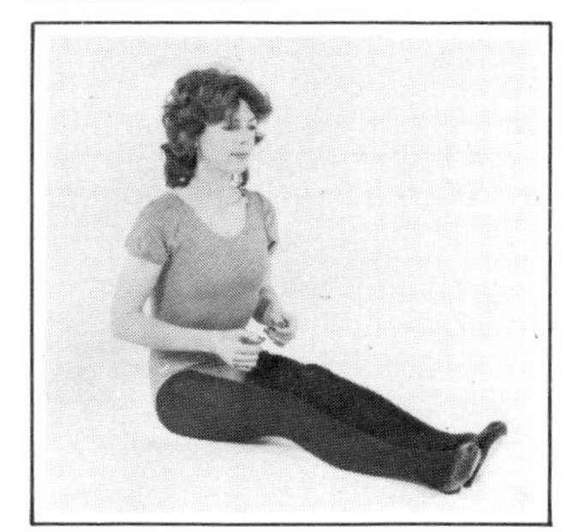

Start Sitting relaxed straight legs, strong back.
▽

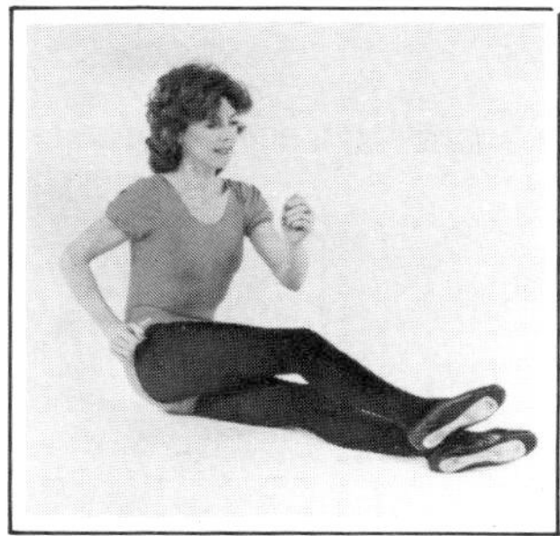

Exercise Walking forwards on bottom then backwards on bottom.
Feel Agile and flexible.
▽

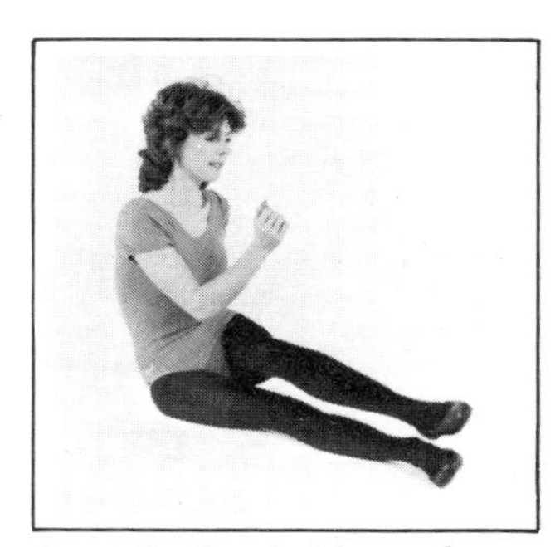

Good For Pelvis, hips and spine.

THE SLIMNASTICS PROGRAMME

Week VII

Healthy Eating Programme (fruit)

This week experiment with fruit. Again you are adding fibre and those vital vitamins and minerals to your diet. You are also giving taste and colour to your meals and cooking which are equally important to satisfy the senses. Buy different and exotic fruits and eat them raw after the main course.

Eat them as quick easy meals and snacks. Cook them with meat, fish, vegetables. Combine them with vegetables for salads. You do not have to spend a great deal of money. One or two fruits can go a long way.

Tension Control Technique (massage)

Continue as before. This week try out the massage technique on p 44. You can either do it by yourself or of course it is much better if someone else can massage your neck, shoulders and back. It can be a soothing and relaxing experience.

Weight this Week .... st. .... lb.

Slimnastics Exercises

Read the Safety Guidelines on p 18.

Wear comfortable clothing. Barefeet or non-slip shoes.

Week VII Do each exercise for 1 minute.

Exercise One

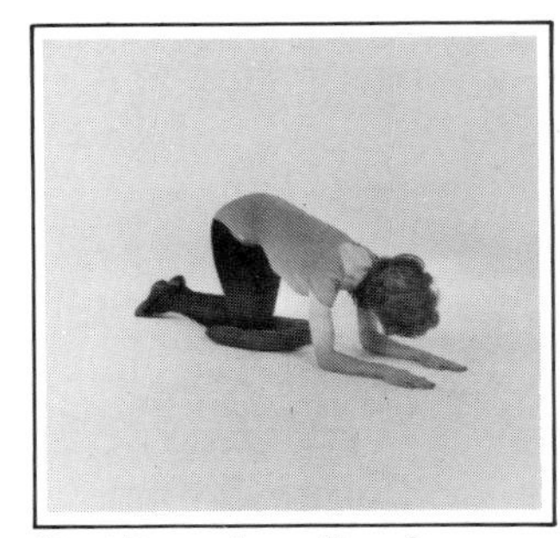

Start Prone kneeling, keep back straight. Elbows under shoulder, knees under hips.
▽

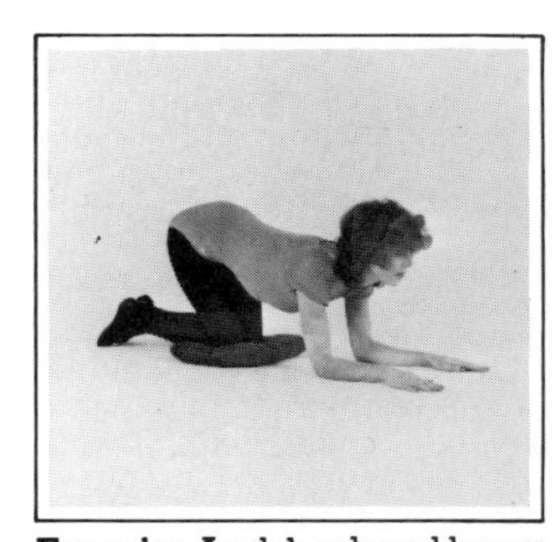

Exercise Arch back and hump back.
Feel Slow movement and flexible spine.
▽

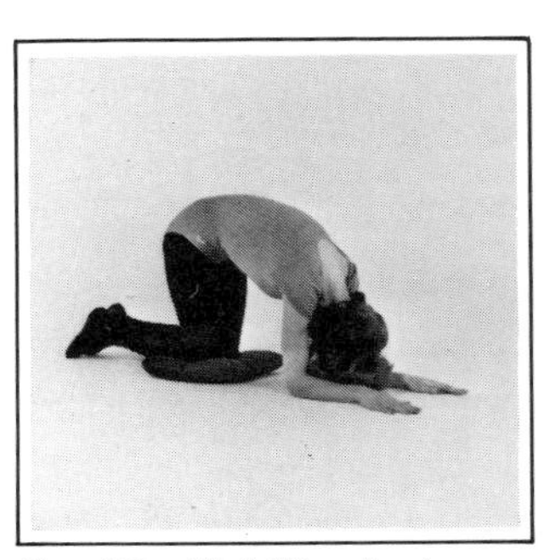

Good For Mobility of spine, waist line.

Exercise Two

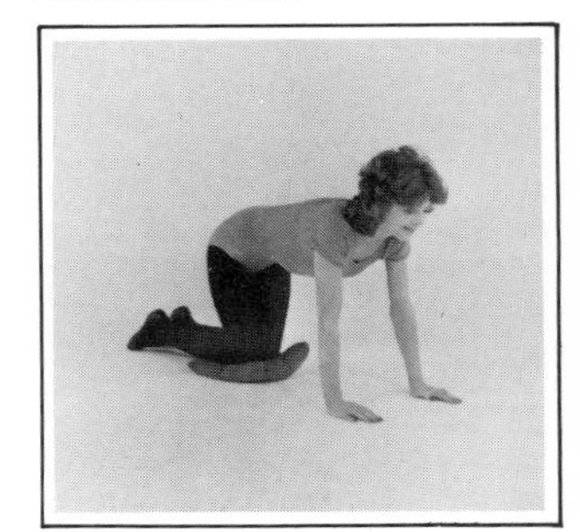

Start Prone kneeling, hands under shoulders, stretch spine.
▽

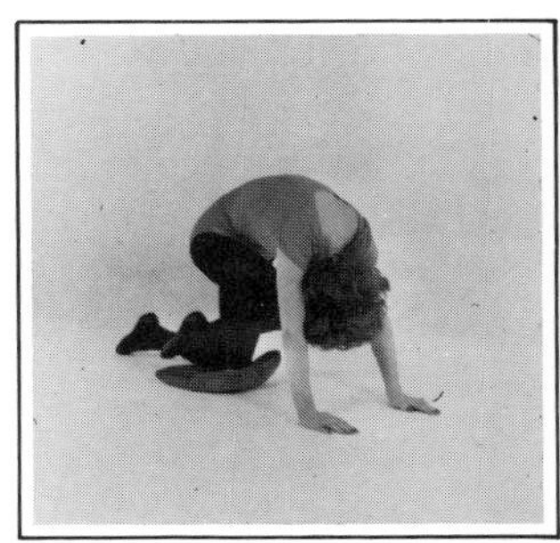

Exercise Bend one leg under body, touch head with knee then stretch leg behind.
Feel Body flexed and slowly stretched.
▽

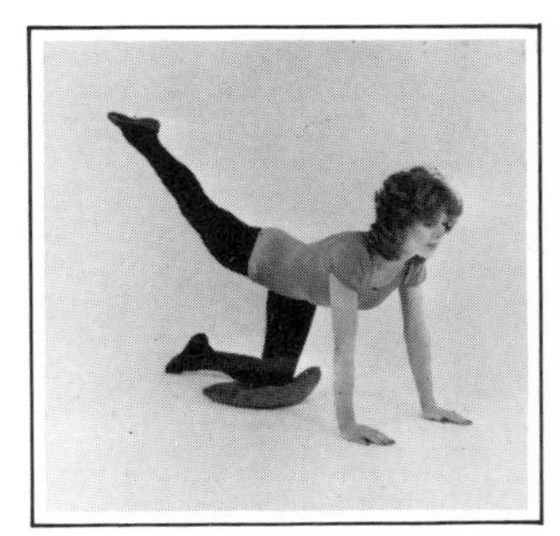

Good For Buttocks and back.

WEEK 7

Exercise Three

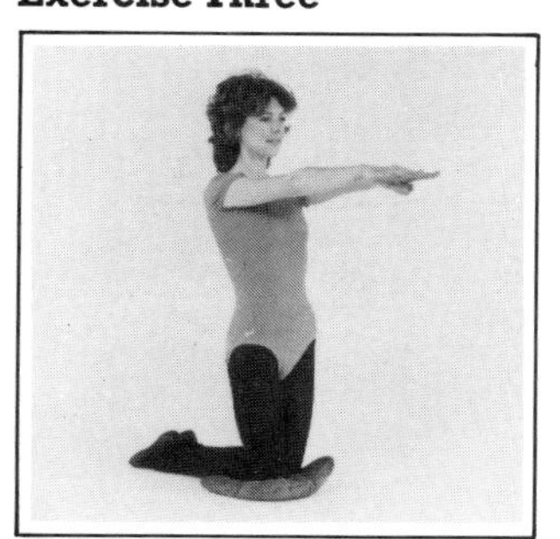

Start Kneeling on cushion. Stretch spine, arms in front.

▽

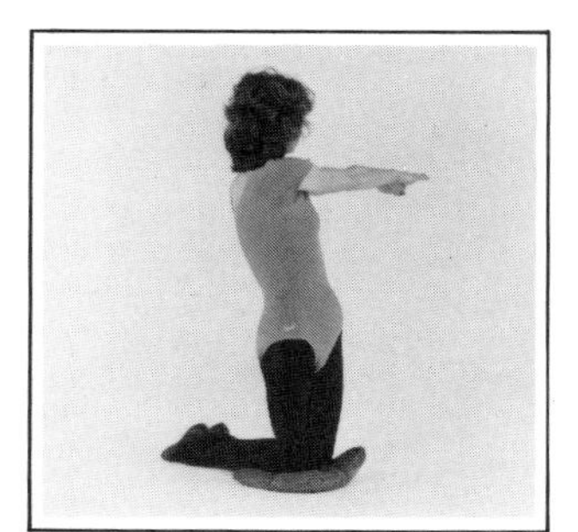

Exercise Turn to one side, then the other.
Feel Spine firm stretched and twisted.

▽

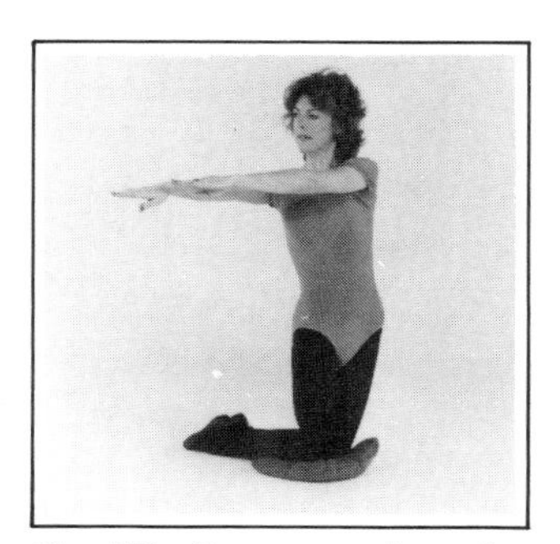

Good For Posture, waist and thighs.

Exercise Four

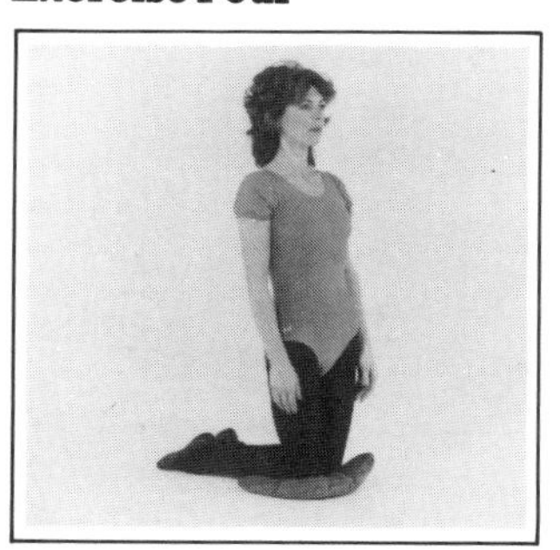

Start Kneeling tall, straight back.

▽

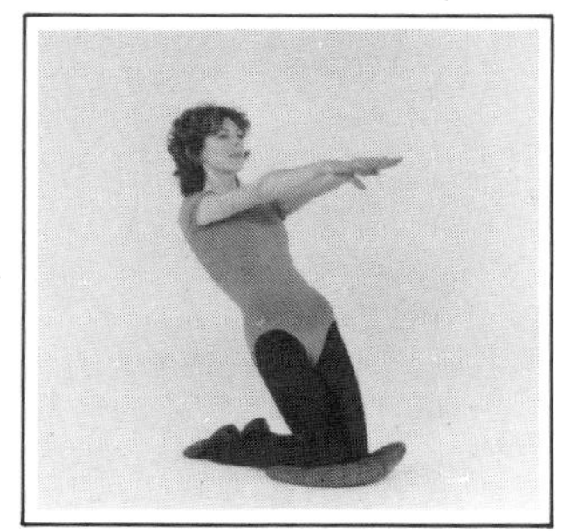

Exercise Lower slowly backwards keeping back and hips straight. Arms come forwards.
Feel Straight from knee to head, movement slow and strong.

▽

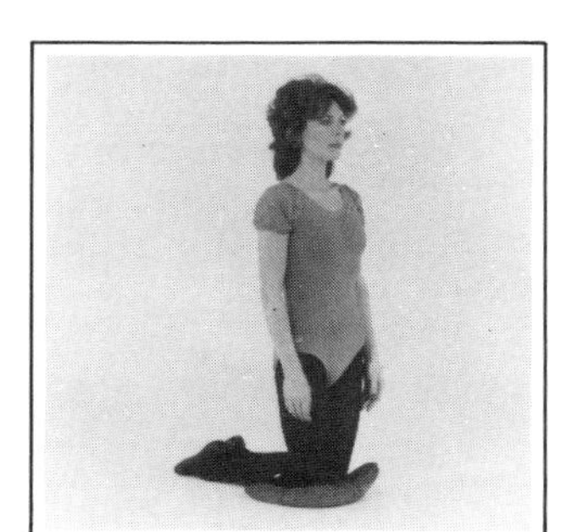

Good For Thighs and abdomen.

Exercise Five

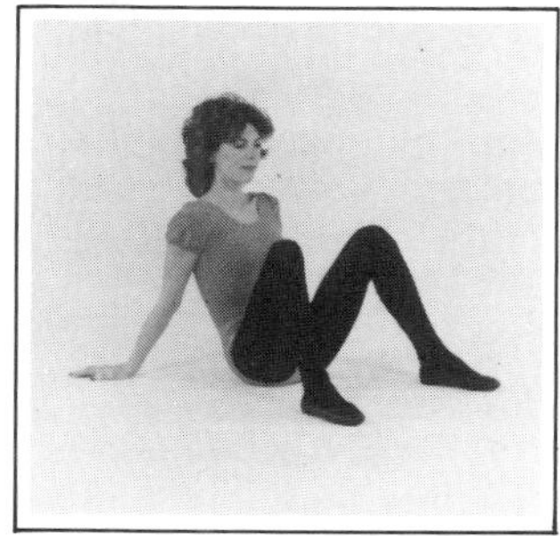

Start Crook sitting with arm support behind. Feet wide apart.

▽

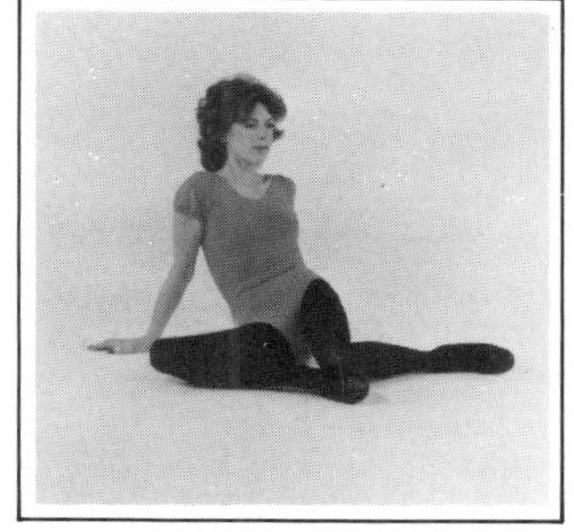

Exercise Lower both knees to floor on the same side, right knee towards left foot. Repeat other side.
Feel Twisted and relaxed.

▽

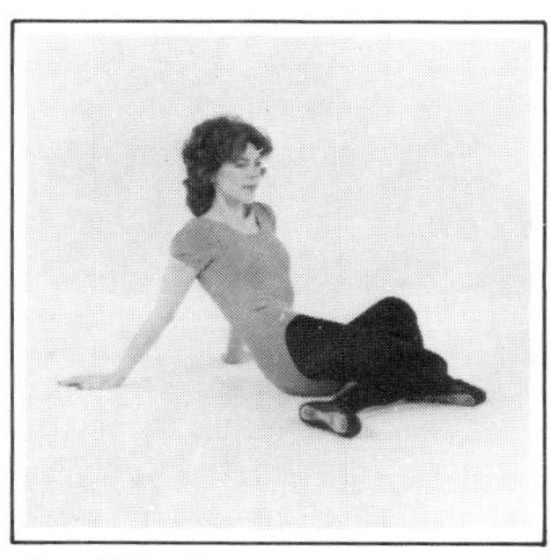

Good For Pelvis, hips and spine.

Exercise Six

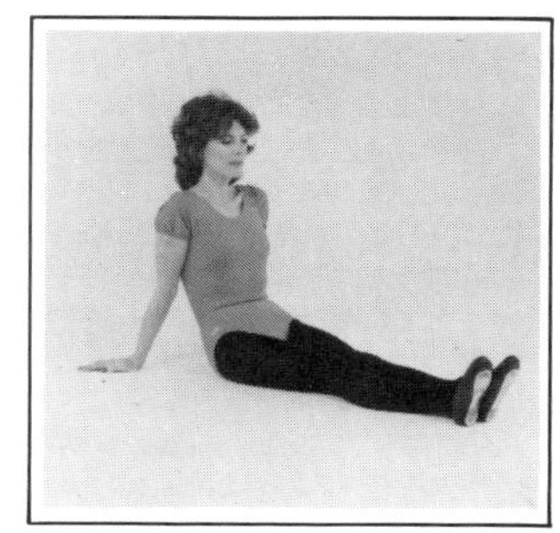

Start Long sitting, straight back, firm knee caps, hands on floor by buttocks.

▽

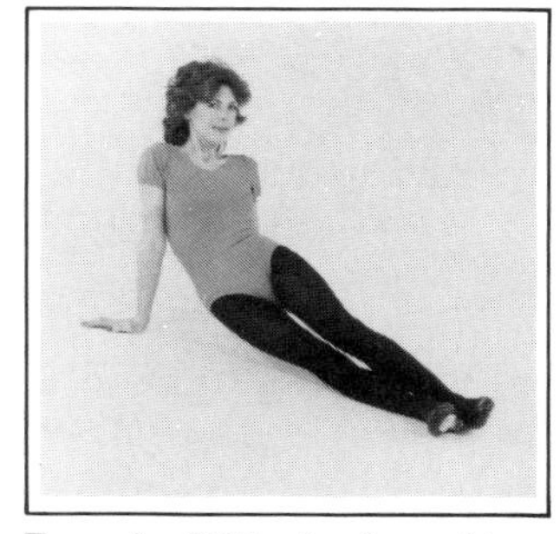

Exercise Lift buttocks and turn body from side to side.
Feel Rhythmical and stretched.

▽

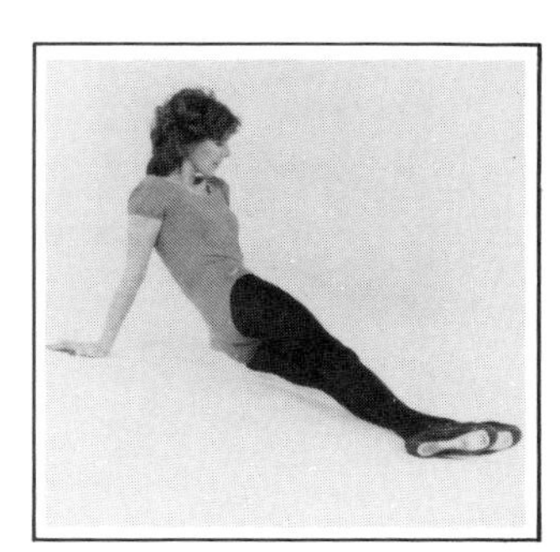

Good For Waist line and spine. Arms and shoulders

THE SLIMNASTICS PROGRAMME

Week VIII
Healthy Eating Programme (herbs)

Your taste buds have more treats in store. This week read the table of herbs in the appendix. We have given the dishes for which they are considered most suitable but there are many more you could try yourself. Of course growing your own herbs makes sure they are at their most nutritious but they are also good to freeze and dried herbs can be excellent (though much stronger so use less in the recipe or you will swamp the other tastes).

Many of our recipes use herbs and you can find others in inexpensive books and magazines.

Tension Control Technique (meditation)

Continue as before. This week try out the Meditation exercise. Remember that if you do it correctly your body will feel completely relaxed but your mind active and alert. This is the time to practise any physical technique you wish to improve – your strokes in swimming, your swing in golf, your aim in darts – you will be surprised how well it works.

Weight this Week .... st. .... lb.

The Slimnastics Exercises

Read the Safety Guidelines on p 18.

Wear comfortable clothing. Barefeet or non-slip shoes.

Week VIII Do each exercise for 1 minute.

Exercise One

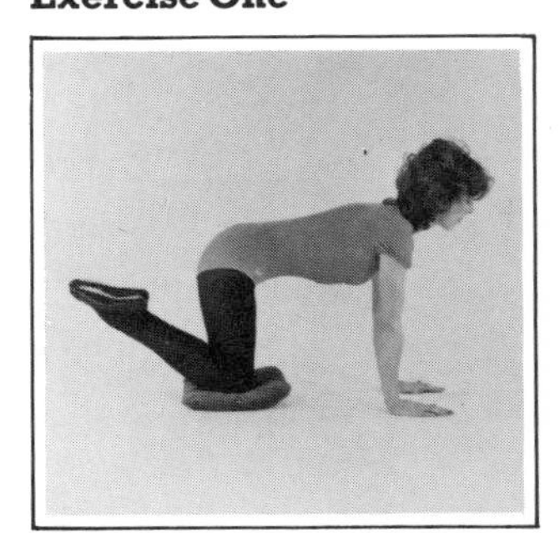

Start Prone kneeling, keep back straight. Elbows under shoulders, knees under hips.

▽

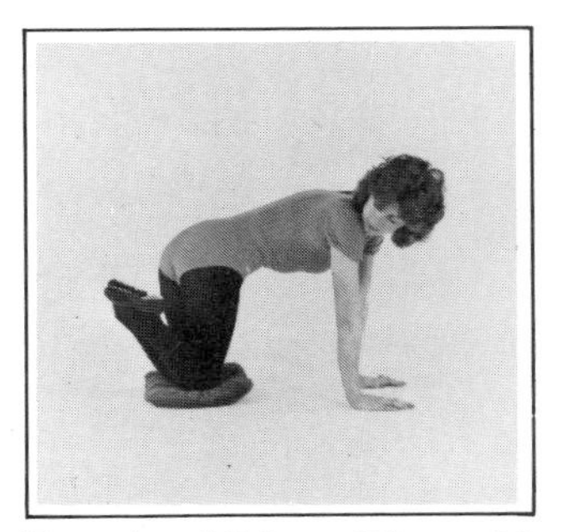

Exercises Lift feet off floor, side bend by moving feet and head to right then left. Circle spine up, side, down, feet on the floor.
Feel Flexibility around the waist.

▽

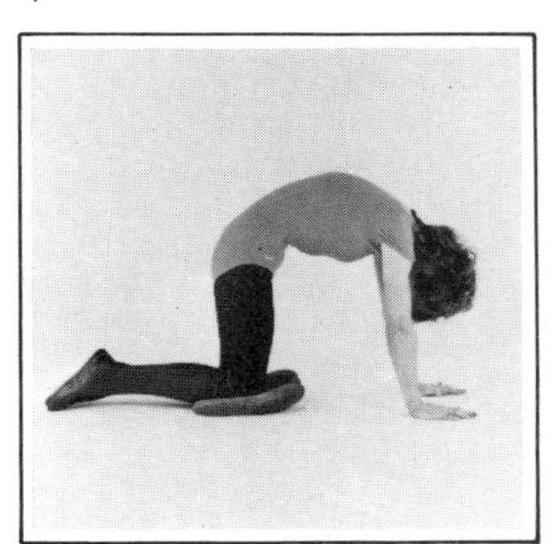

Good For Spine and back mobility.

Exercise Two

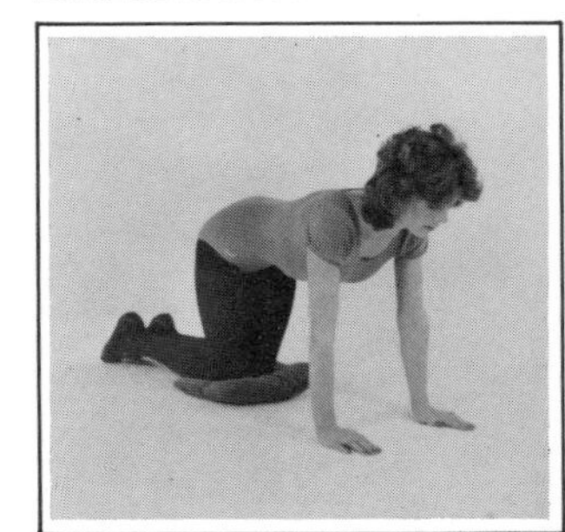

Start Prone kneeling, hands under shoulders, stretched spine.

▽

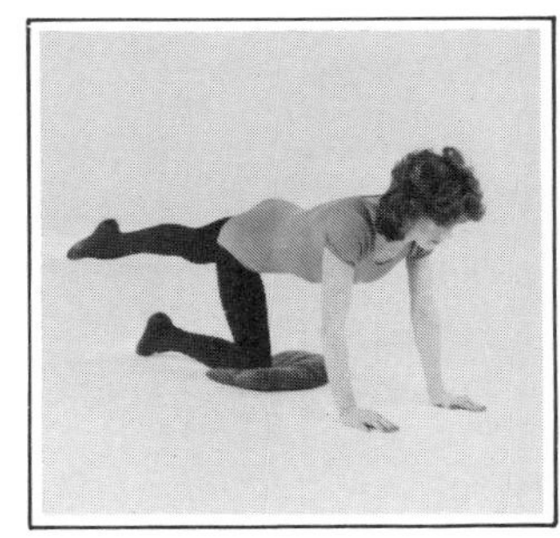

Exercise Straight leg behind, lift up and down, then circle. Repeat with other leg.
Feel Strength and mobility.

▽

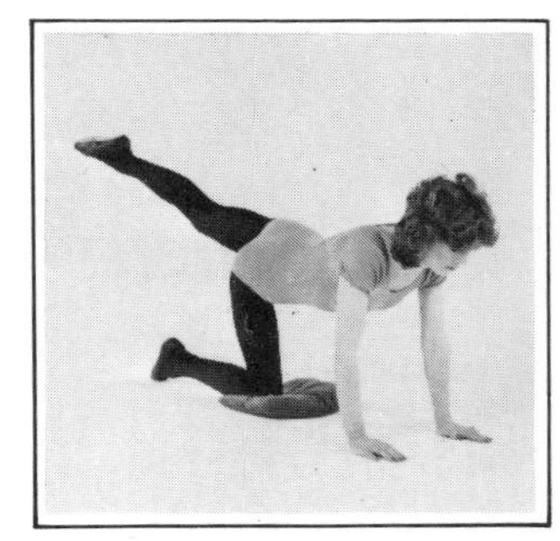

Good For Back, buttocks, thigh.

WEEK 8

Exercise Three

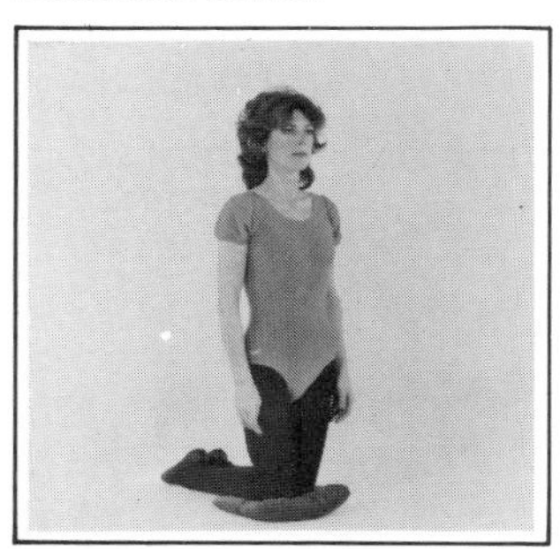

Start Kneeling on cushion. Stretch spine. Arms by sides.
▽

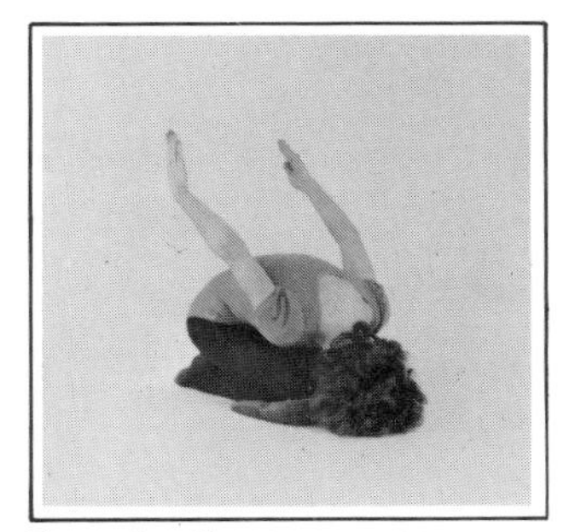

Exercise Curl body with arms behind back then stretch up tall, arms above head.
Feel Curled and stretched tall.
▽

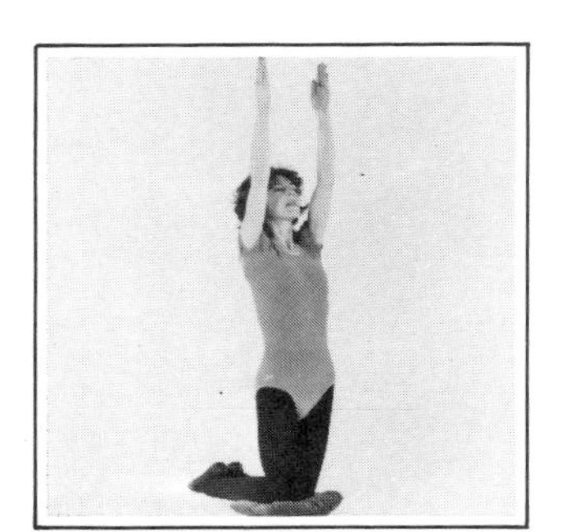

Good For Thighs, hips, arms and shoulders.

Exercise Four

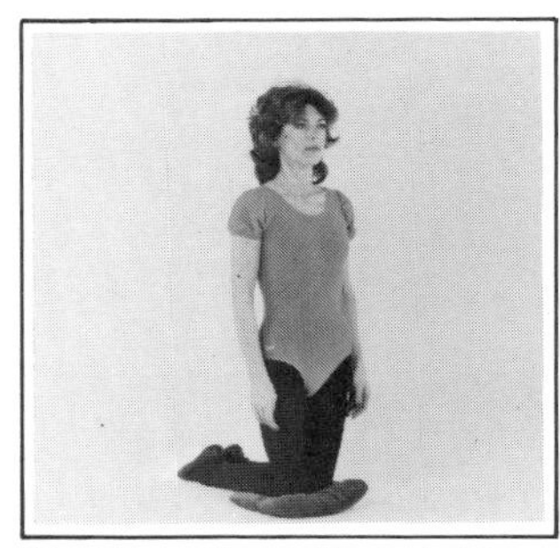

Start Kneeling tall, straight back.
▽

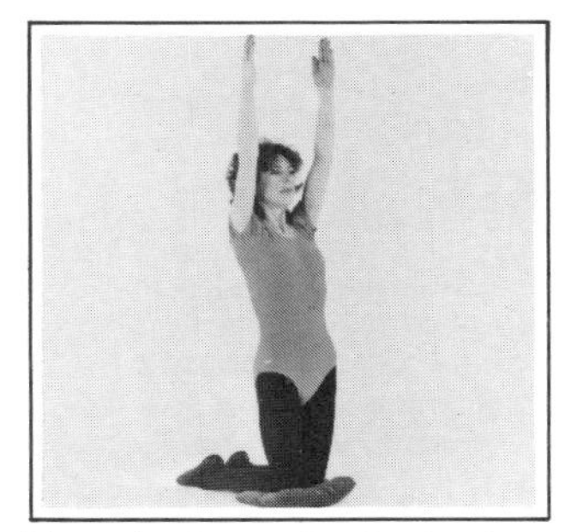

Exercise Lower body slowly backwards keeping back and hips straight and raise both arms sideways. Raise body and stretch arms above head.
Feel Strong and straight back and stomach; stretched arms and shoulders.
▽

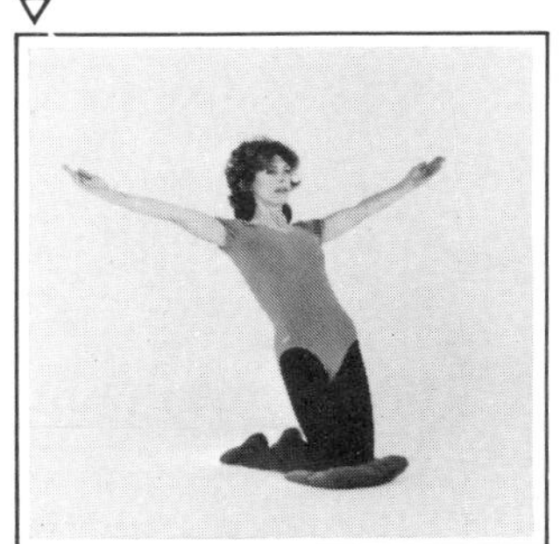

Good For Tummy and thighs.

Exercise Five

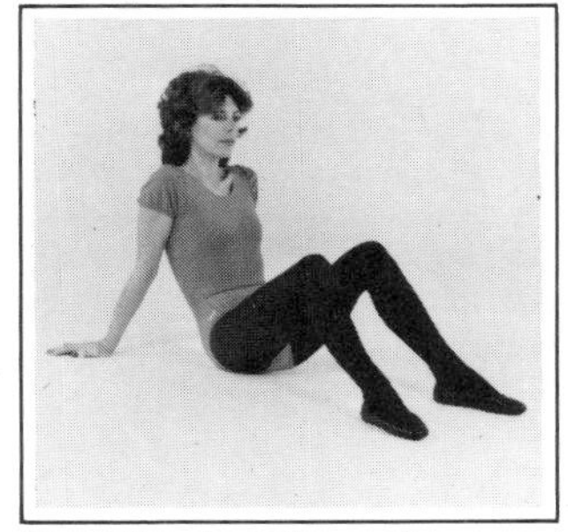

Start Crook sitting with arm support behind. Legs wide apart.
▽

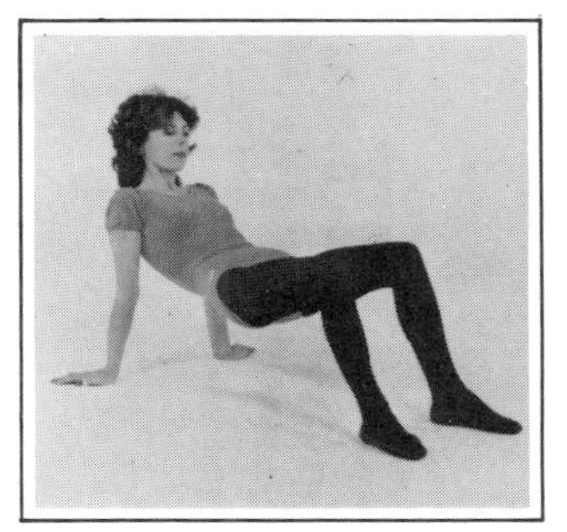

Exercise Lift hips off floor. Harden buttocks, squeeze pelvic floor muscles. Don't arch spine.
Feel Firm, slow continuous movement.

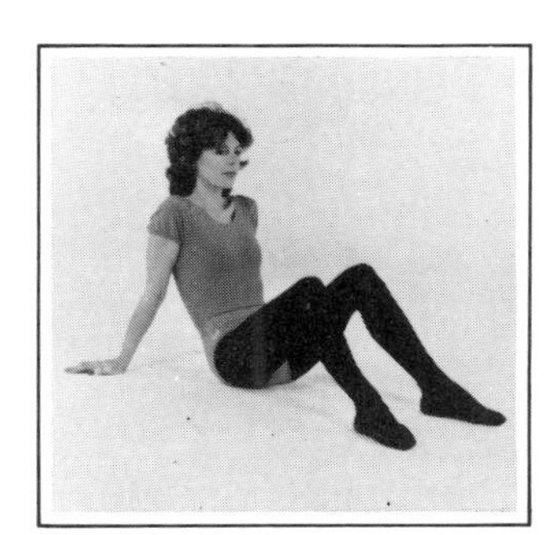

Good For Back, arms and buttocks.

Exercise Six

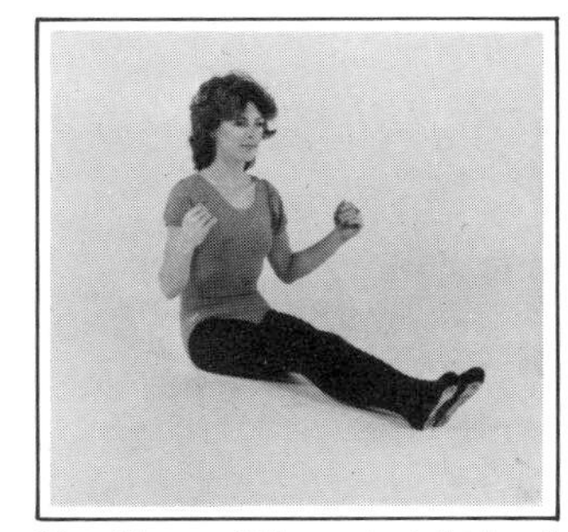

Start Long sitting, straight back. Bent arms in front at shoulder level.

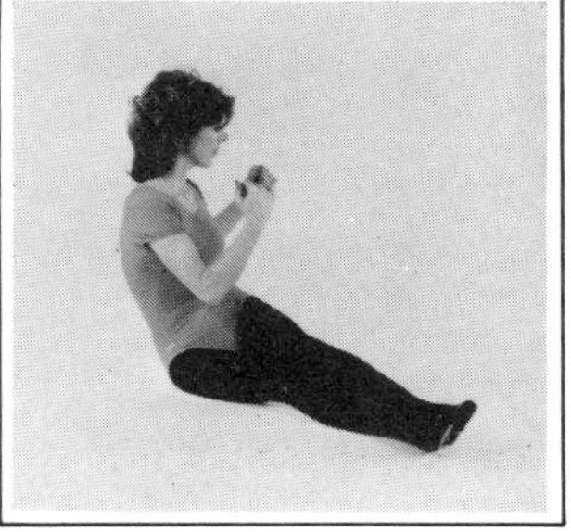

Exercise Turn to one side, lift same buttock. Repeat other side.
Feel Rhythmical exercise, relaxed knees.
▽

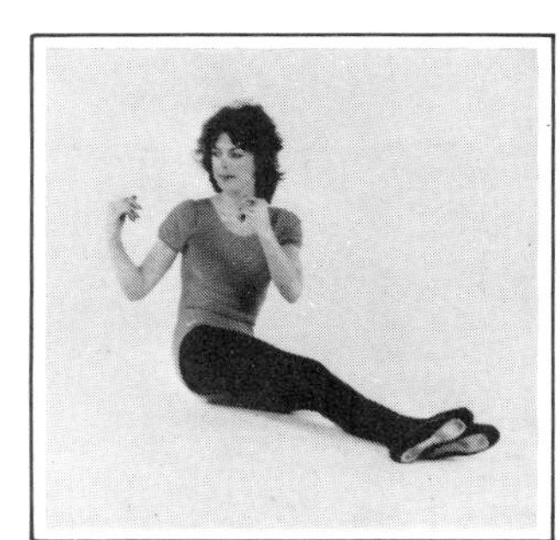

Good For Waist, spine.

THE SLIMNASTICS PROGRAMME

Week IX

Healthy Eating Programme (spices)

Luckily with so many more ethnic restaurants and shops we are beginning to be more aware and used to different spices and tastes. They are also more readily available in our shops. We have given you a list of their more usual uses (confining it to the most healthy dishes) but you may know more. This week concentrate on using more of these. Use them discreetly until you establish how much is right for you and your family. We use several in our recipes and there are many more ideas to be found in magazines and inexpensive cookery books.

Tension Control Technique (sleep)

Continue as before. Practise the sleep exercises this week just before you fall asleep each night. You may have no difficulty sleeping at this moment but we all have times when we are overtired, our lives are so full, or we have worries, anxieties or problems when getting to sleep, or waking in the night becomes an extra burden in itself. Mastering this technique so that you can use it when such an occasion arises is a blessing; it does take some concentration and practise so it is worth doing when you are able to give it some thought.

Weight this Week .... st. .... lb.

The Slimnastics Exercises

Read the Safety Guidelines on p 18.

Wear comfortable clothing. Barefeet or non-slip shoes.

Week IX Do each exercise for 1 minute.

Exercise One

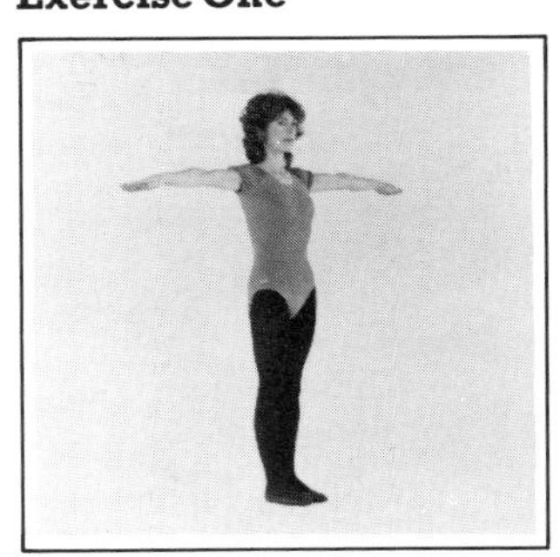

Start Stand tall, long neck, arms out at shoulder level.

▽

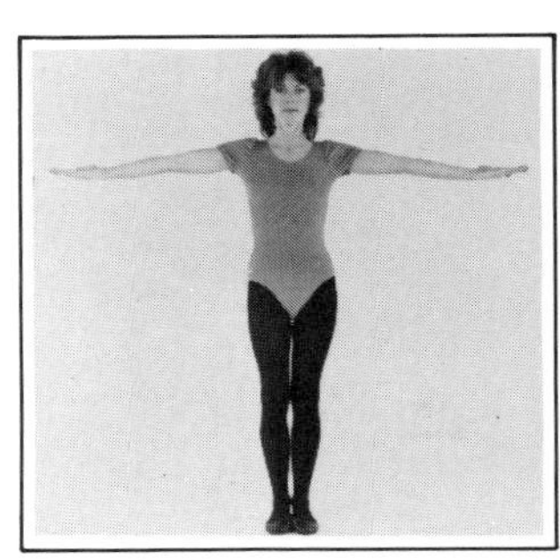

Exercise Rotate arms, palms facing upwards and then backs of hands facing downwards.
Feel Strong, medium-paced exercise. Stretch posture.

▽

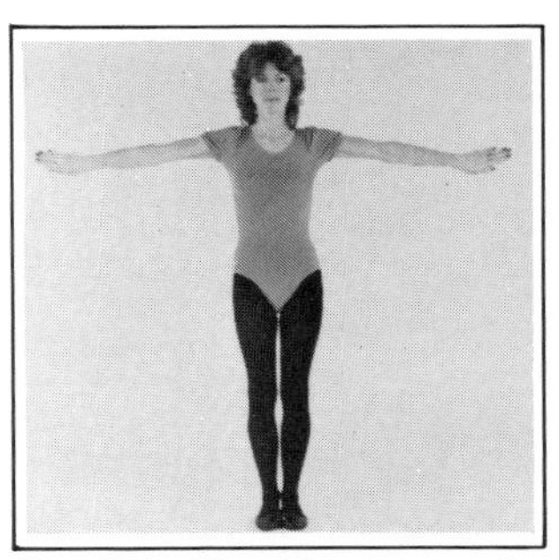

Good For Shoulder joint and arms.

Exercise Two

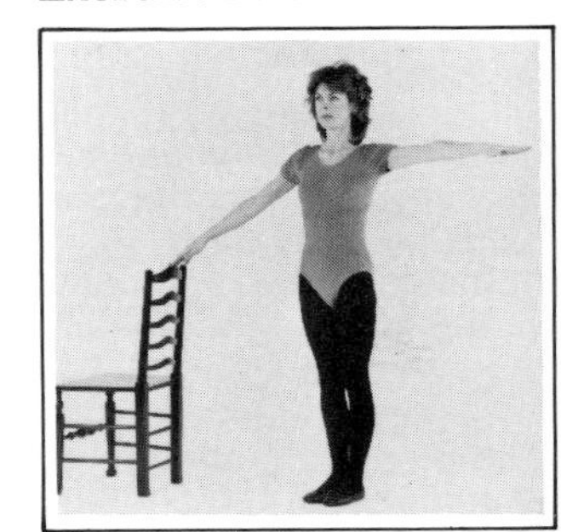

Start Stand tall with hand lightly on a chair to balance.

▽

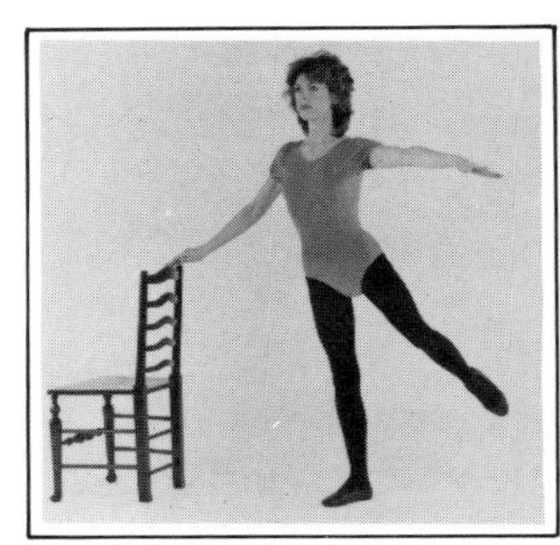

Exercise Swing outside leg forwards and backwards.
Feel Balanced and easy.

▽

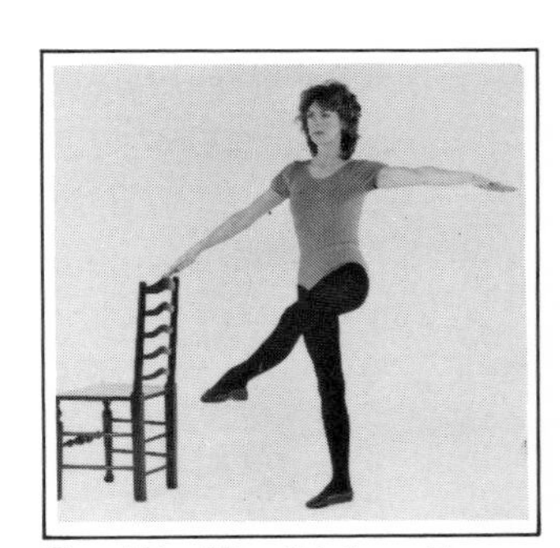

Good For Hip, thigh and leg.

WEEK 9

Exercise Three

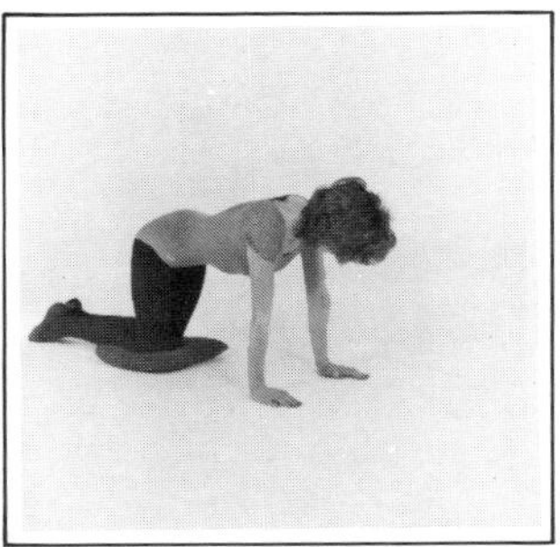

Start Prone kneeling, hands under shoulders, knees under hips.
▽

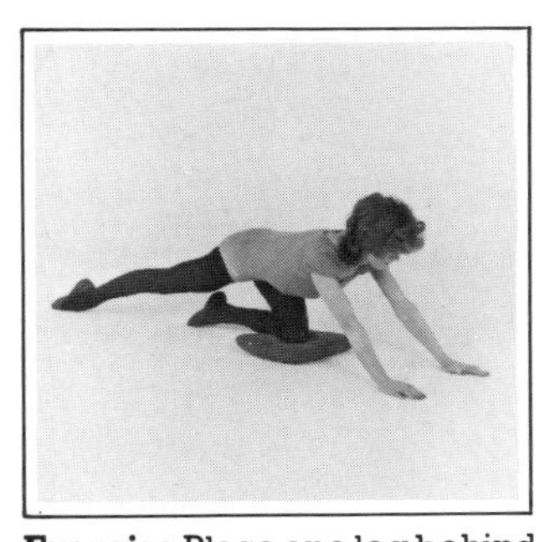

Exercise Place one leg behind. Move slowly backwards to full stretch of arms and leg.
Feel Strong, slow and stretched.
▽

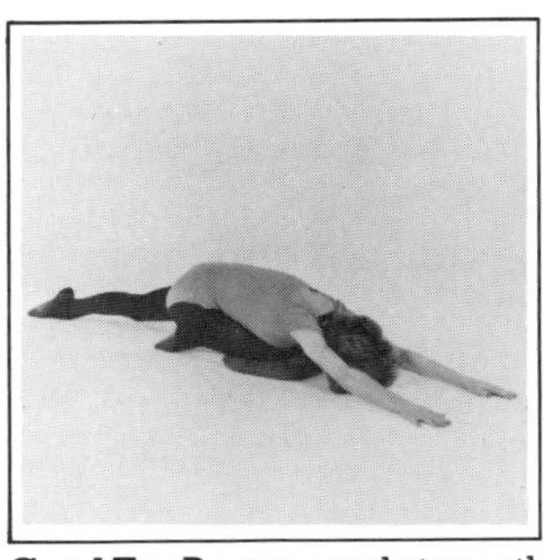

Good For Posture and strength of whole body.

Exercise Four

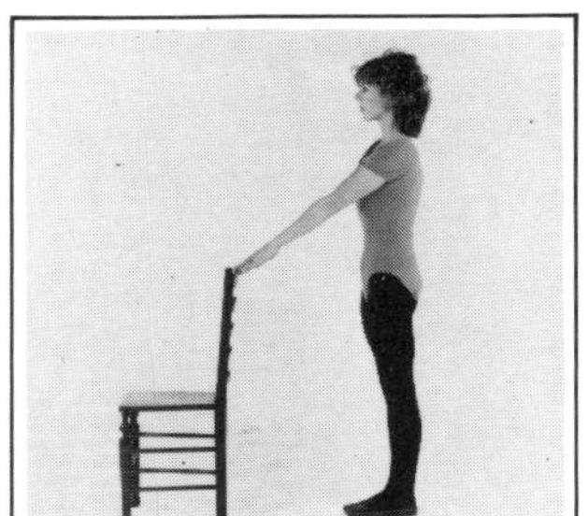

Start Standing tall, facing chair, relaxed shoulders.
▽

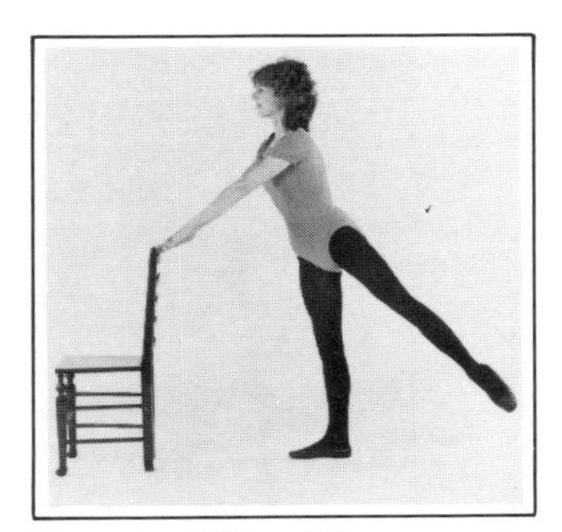

Exercise Lift back leg up and down, toe pointed (with knee facing outwards).
Feel Body stretched and tall, continuous movement.
▽

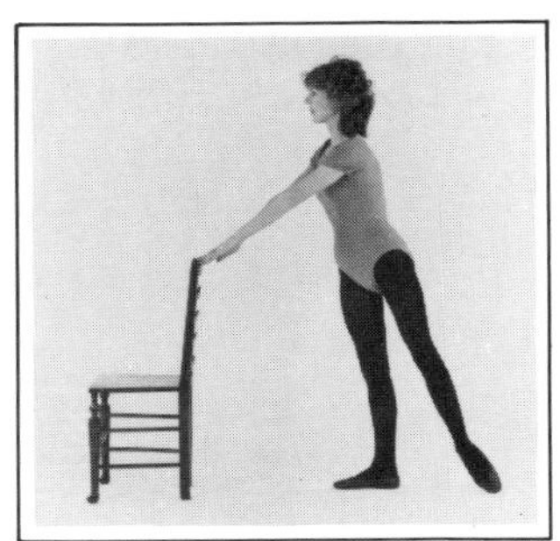

Good For Buttocks, posture and lower back.

Exercise Five

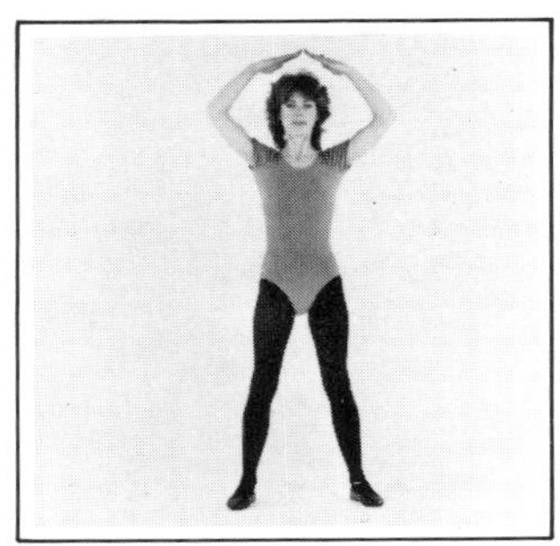

Start Standing tall, feet apart, hands lightly above head, long neck.
▽

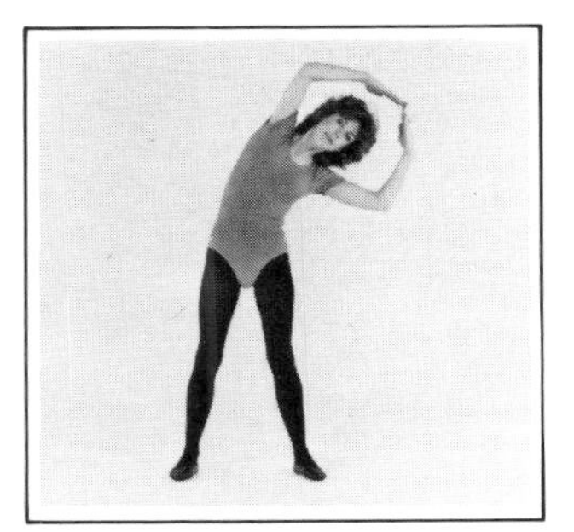

Exercise Bend to alternate sides.
Feel Firm, stretched and balanced.
▽

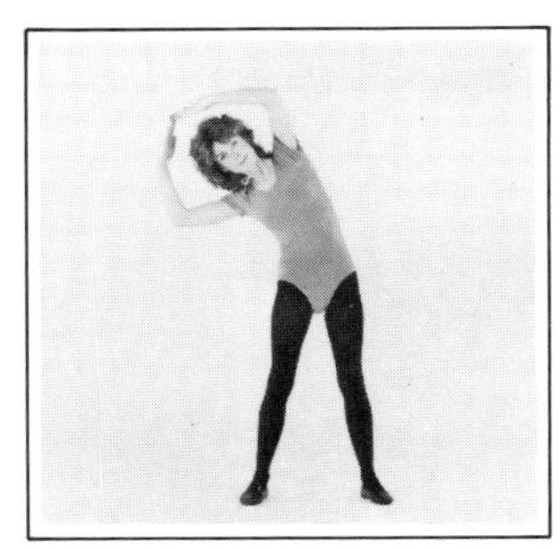

Good For Waist line and back.

Exercise Six

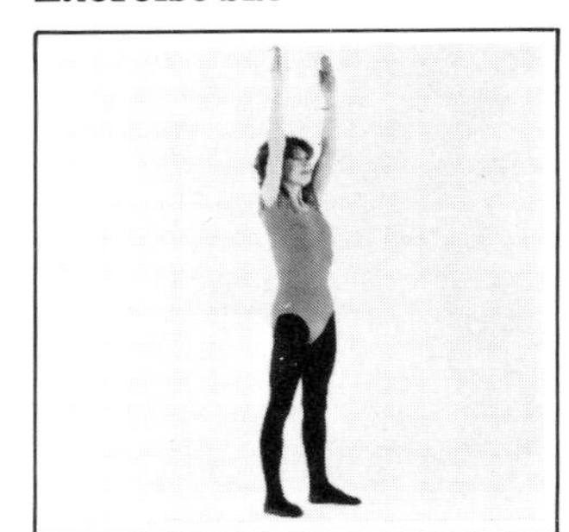

Start Stand tall, legs apart. Arms stretched above head.
▽

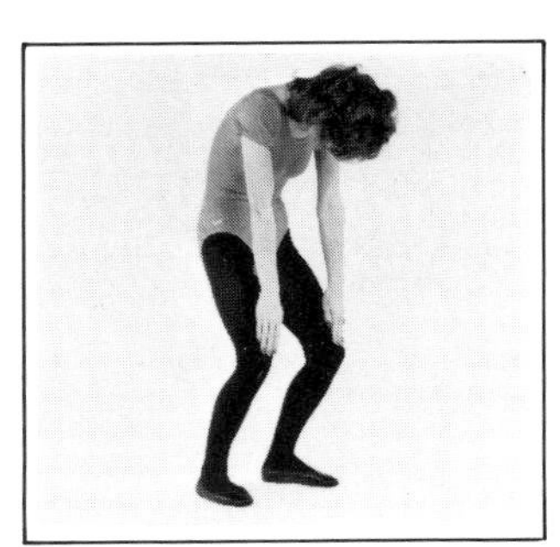

Exercise Bend legs, touch knees, then stretch tall. Arms above head, legs straight.
Feel Relaxed and then stretched.
▽

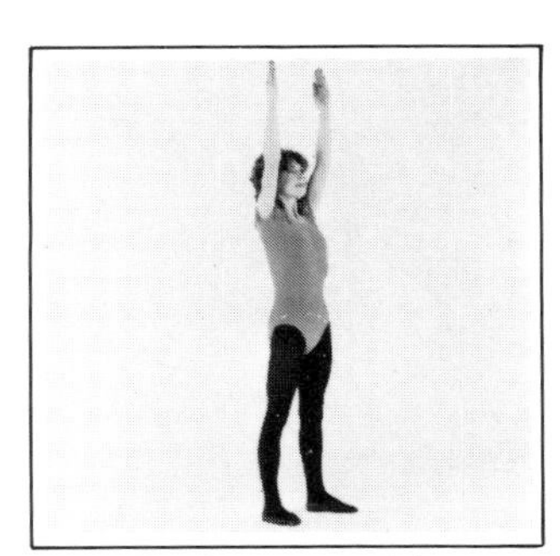

Good For Stretching joints gently.

THE SLIMNASTICS PROGRAMME

Week X
Healthy Eating Programme (fluids)

This week make a note of all your fluid intake. Jot down every cup of coffee, tea, water, mineral water, fruit juice and also write down your alcohol intake.

At the end of the week see how much caffeine and tannin you consume (in the tea and coffee), how many calories in the fruit juice (think how many fruits it takes to squeeze that amount and remember if you had the whole fruit you would have the fibre too!) and count the units of alcohol (p 52). You need at least 5 pints of water a day (some of it in fruit and vegetables). You do not *need* any alcohol. Over 6 units harms the health of a man, over 3 units is unsafe for a woman.

Tension Control Technique (use time well)

Continue as before. Read the first chapter in Section 4 and decide how you can make best use of your time. Decide if there are more ways in which you can find time to yourself even if it is only daydreaming on the bus on the way to work, listening to the radio or joining a Slimnastics Group or reputable exercise class.

Time to yourself is well spent.

Weight this Week .... st. .... lb.

The Slimnastics Exercises

Read the Safety Guidelines on p 18.

Wear comfortable clothing. Barefeet or non-slip shoes.

Week X Do each exercise for 1 minute.

Exercise One

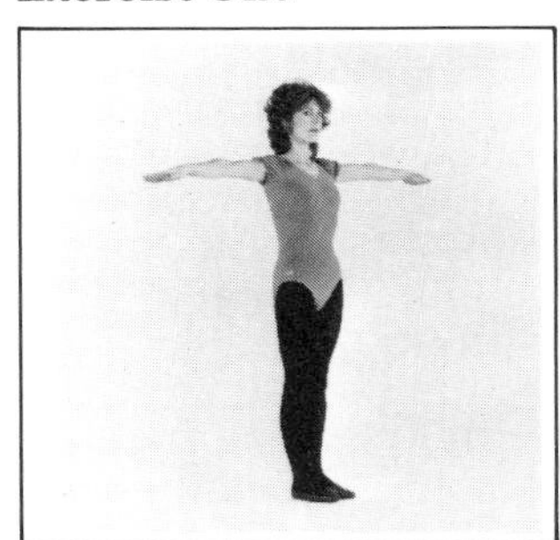

Start Stand tall, long neck, arms and shoulders level, palms facing downwards, relaxed shoulders.
▽

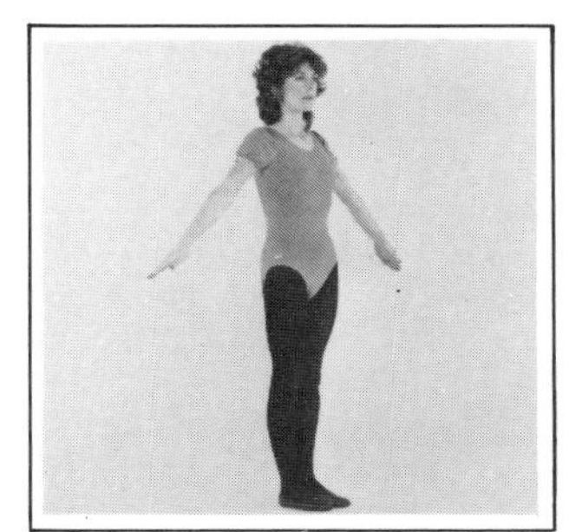

Exercise Keeping arms straight, circle whole arm one way then the other.
Feel Stretched posture, easy movement.
▽

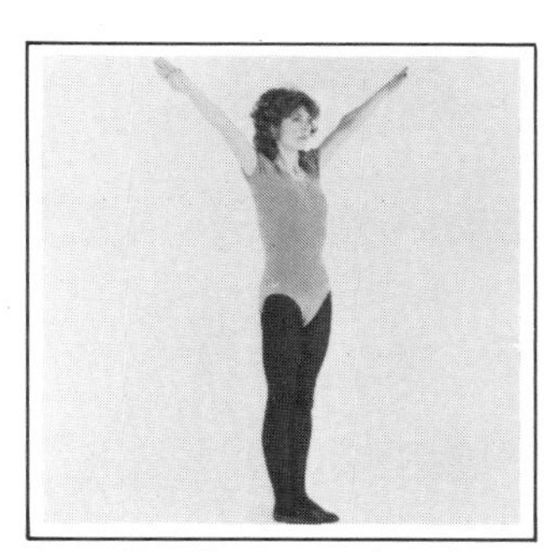

Good For Upper back and shoulders.

Exercise Two

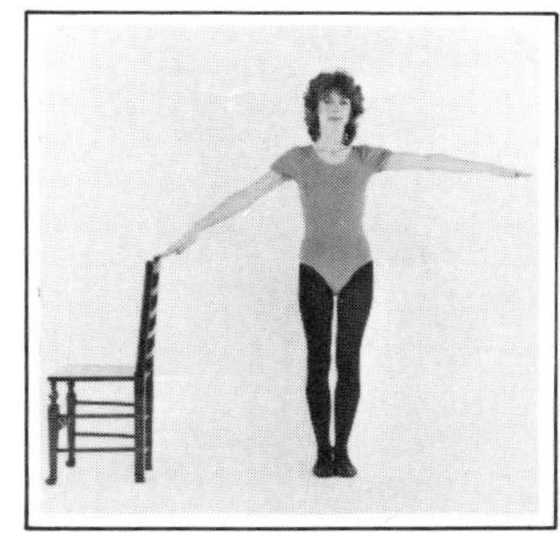

Start Stand tall with hand lightly on chair to balance.
▽

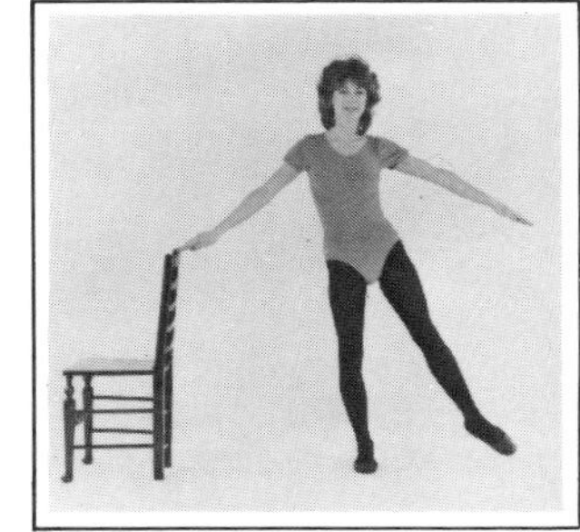

Exercise Circle outside leg anti-clockwise then clockwise. Keep body straight and stretched tall.
Feel Balanced posture and circling movement sideways.
▽

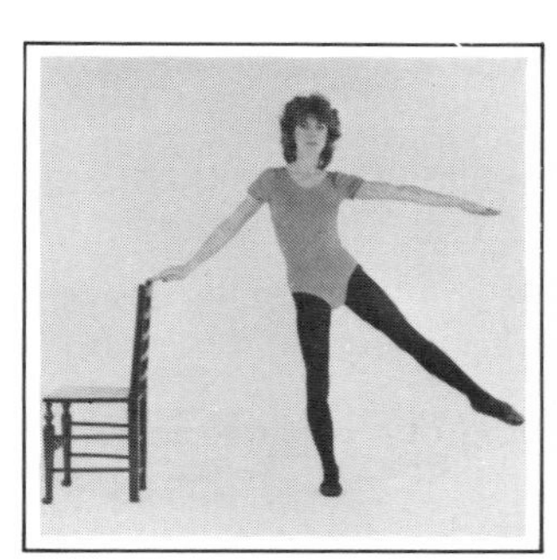

Good For Outside thigh and legs in general.

WEEK 10

Exercise Three

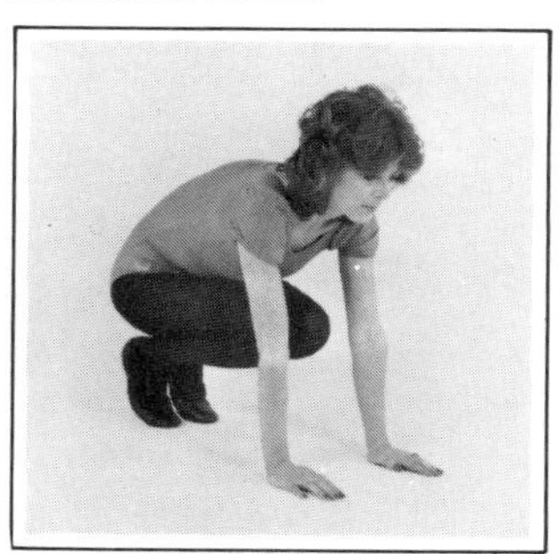

Start Crouch support, hands under shoulders, feet under hips.

▽

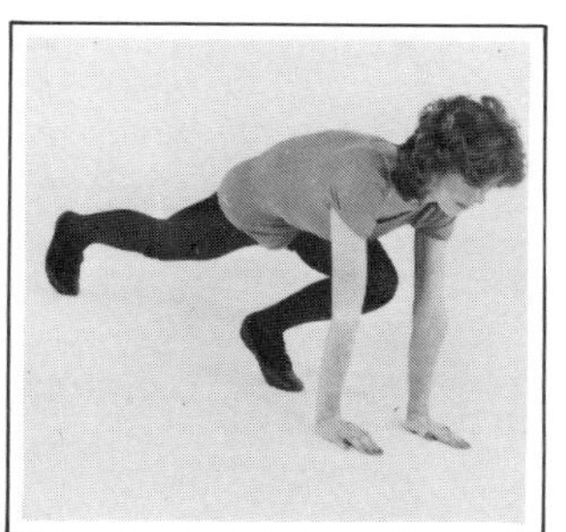

Exercise Place one leg out behind, press hips towards floor, keep tummy firm and back straight.
Feel Strong slow exercise; stretched hips.

▽

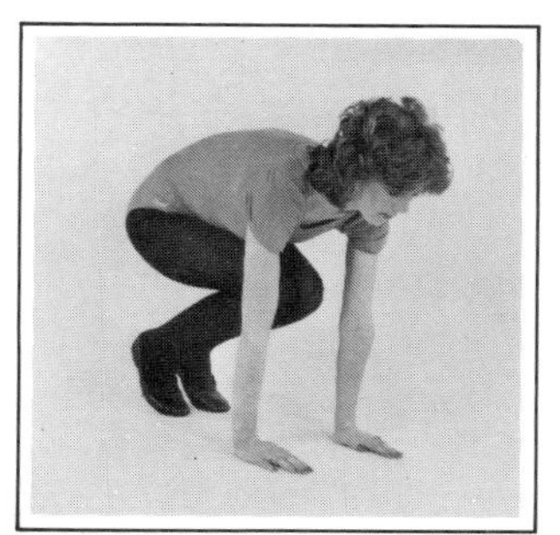

Good For Abdominals, hips and legs.

Exercise Four

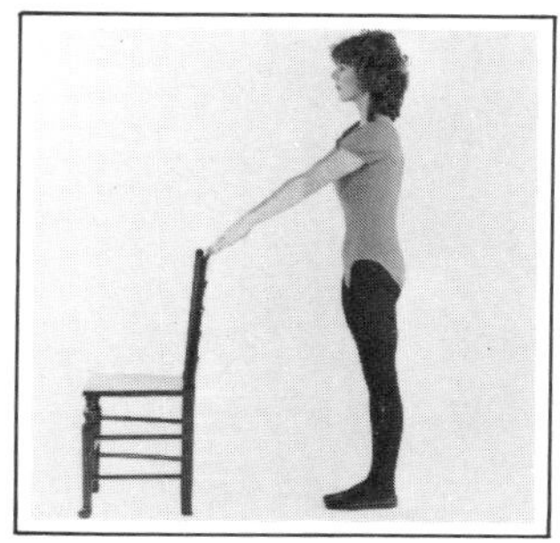

Start Standing tall facing support, keep back straight.

▽

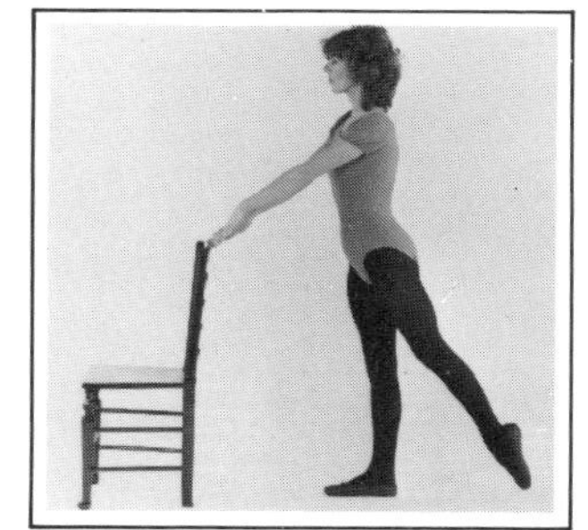

Exercise Lift one leg behind, circle it first one way then the other.
Feel Stretched and tall posture, circling movement behind.

▽

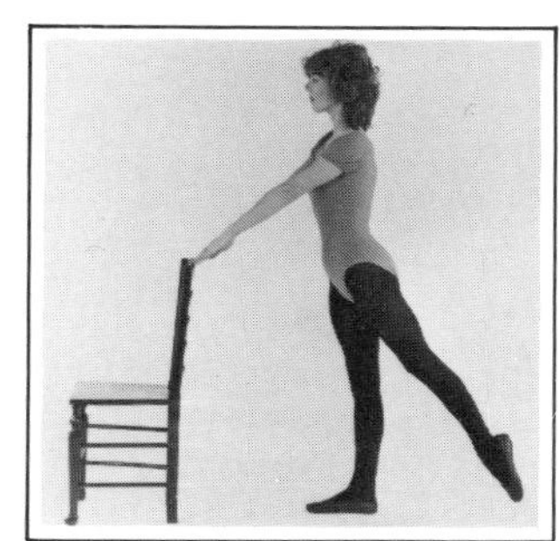

Good For Posture, lower back and buttocks.

Exercise Five

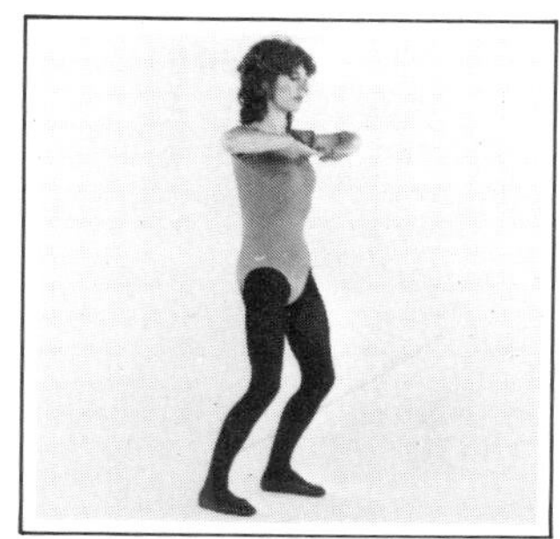

Start Standing tall, feet apart, thighs firm, knees slightly bent. Arms bent at shoulder level in front of chest.

▽

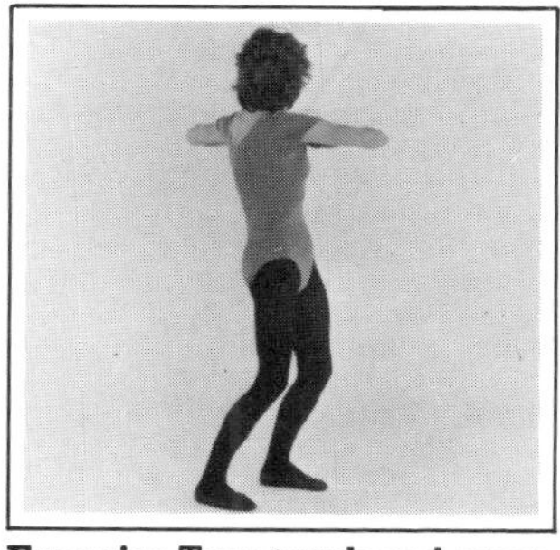

Exercise Turn trunk and arms to alternate sides. Hips and knees face front.
Feel Firm and balanced.

▽

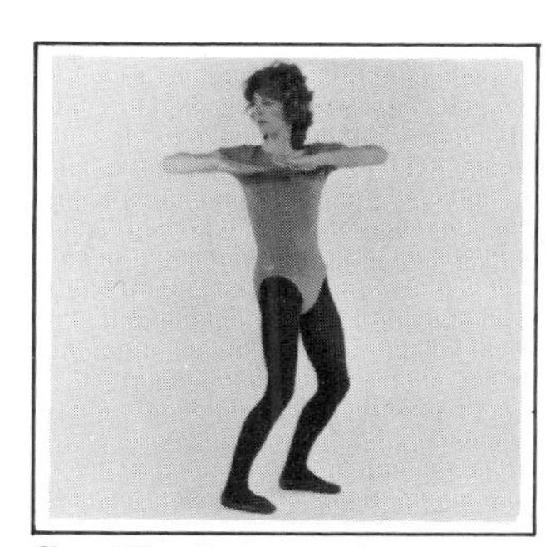

Good For Spine, waist, arms and shoulders.

Exercise Six

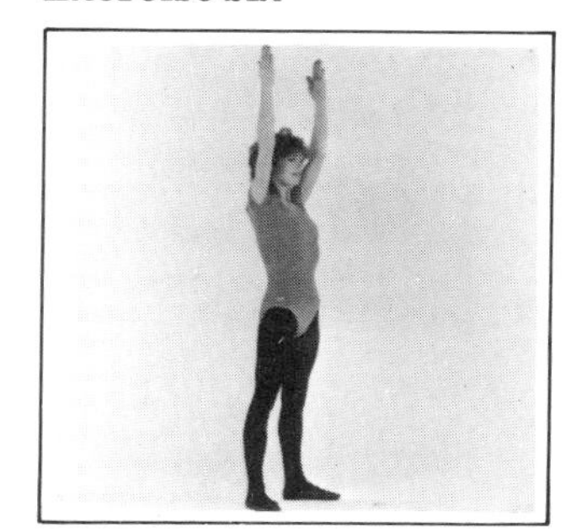

Start Stand tall, legs apart. Arms stretched above head.

▽

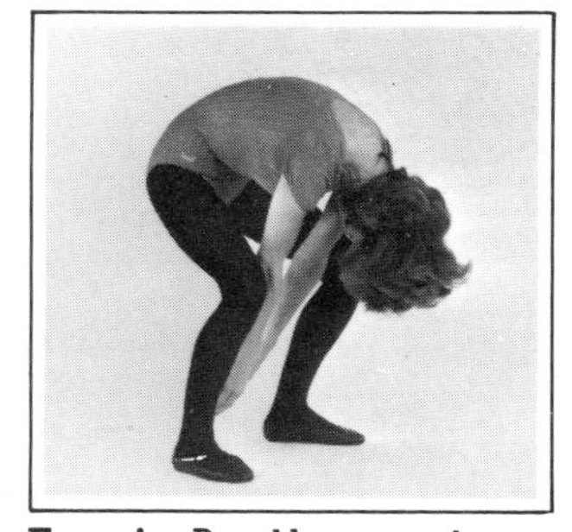

Exercise Bend knees, relax back, reach towards floor.
Feel Relaxed and stretched.

▽

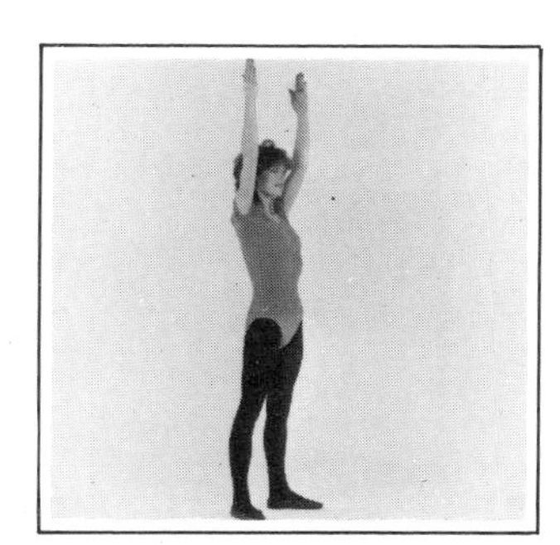

Good For Stretching and mobility.

THE SLIMNASTICS PROGRAMME

Week XI

Healthy Eating Programme (healthy menus)

Buy the foods for one of the suggested menus on pp 38-9 and stick to it for one week. With both, allow yourself only half a pint of skimmed milk a day and 2/3 pieces of fresh fruit. You can have as much water or mineral water as you like but try to have at least 4½ pints.

Tension Control Technique (life events)

Continue as before. Go on planning your use of time by thinking of holidays or events in the next few months, putting them in your diary ensuring they do not overlap and that you are not in danger of overcrowding your Life Events. If your life is short of events manufacture a few more which you will really find possible and able to carry out – visit an old friend, make a new one, go to a concert, help in a charity shop, the possibilities are endless, need a little confidence but are well worth while if you can do them regularly.

Weight this Week .... st. .... lb.

The Slimnastics Exercises

Read the Safety Guidelines on p 18.

Wear comfortable clothing. Barefeet or non-slip shoes.

Week XI Do each exercise for 1 minute.

Exercise One

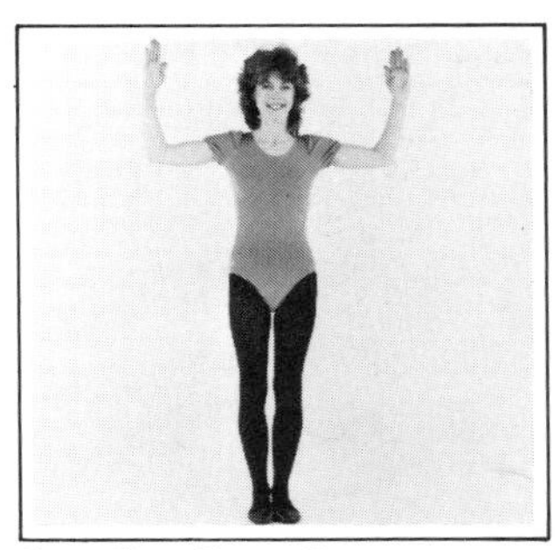

Start Standing tall, upper arms at shoulder level.
▽

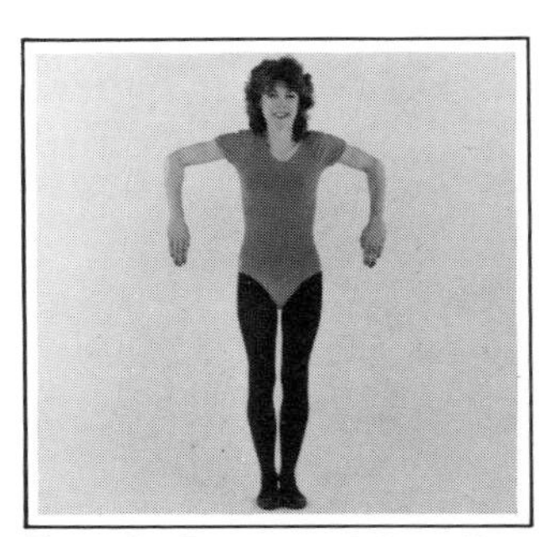

Exercise Lower and then lift forearms and head up.
Feel Slow exercise with strong rotation.
▽

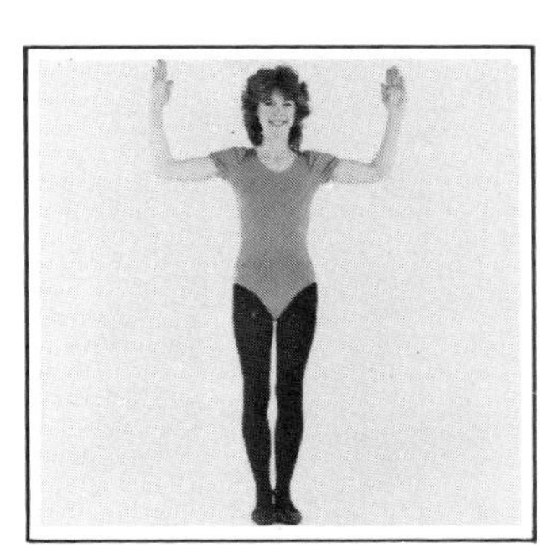

Good For Shoulder joint and arms.

Exercise Two

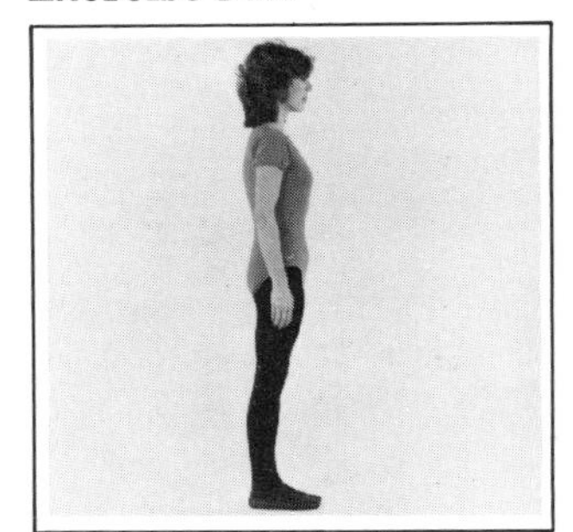

Start Stand tall and firm.
▽

Exercise Lift one knee and hold tight. Balance (or hop – your choice). Change legs.
Feel Balanced posture, stretched joints.
▽

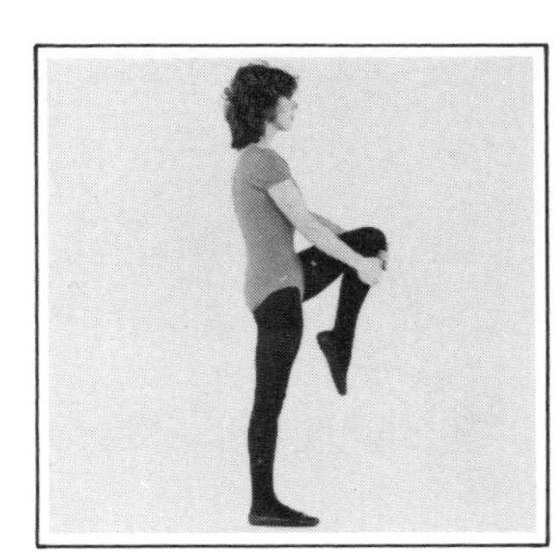

Good For Co-ordination.

WEEK 11

Exercise Three

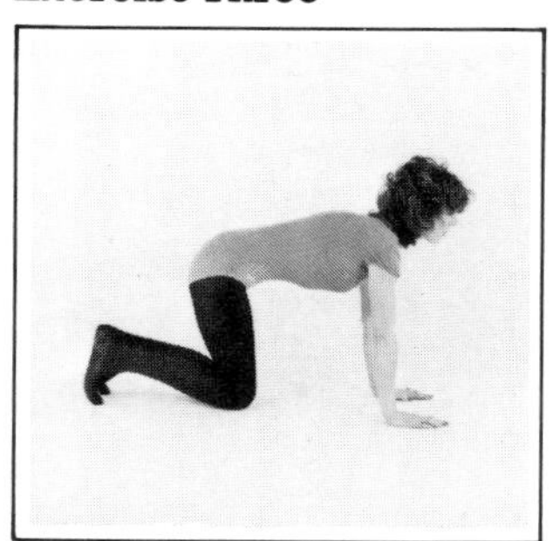

Start Prone kneeling, hands under shoulders, knees under hips.
▽

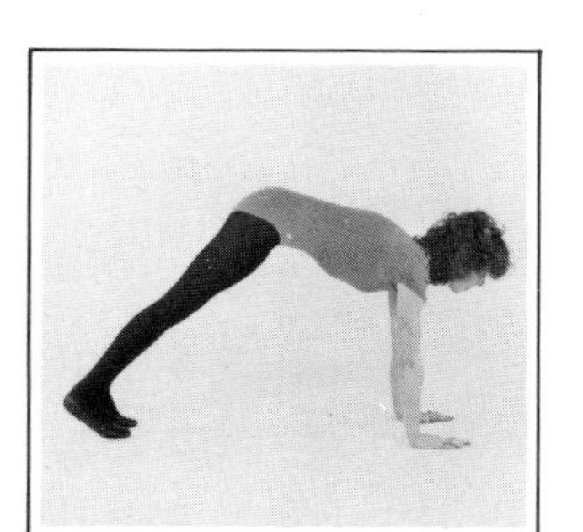

Exercise Lift hips, gently press one heel into floor at a time – bend other knee.
Feel Strong arms and trunk; rhythmical movement of legs.
▽

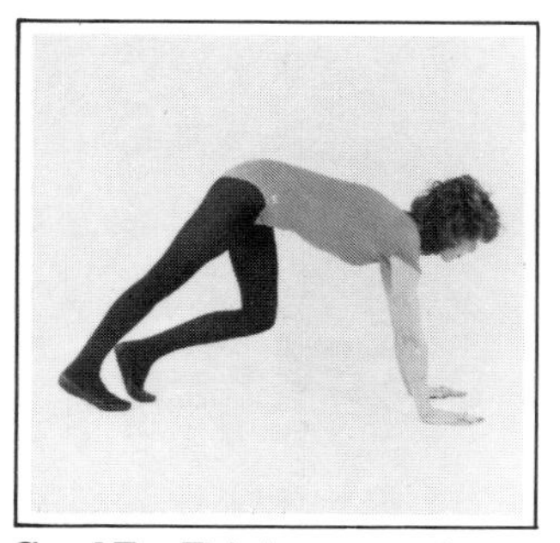

Good For Thighs, stomach, arms and legs.

Exercise Four

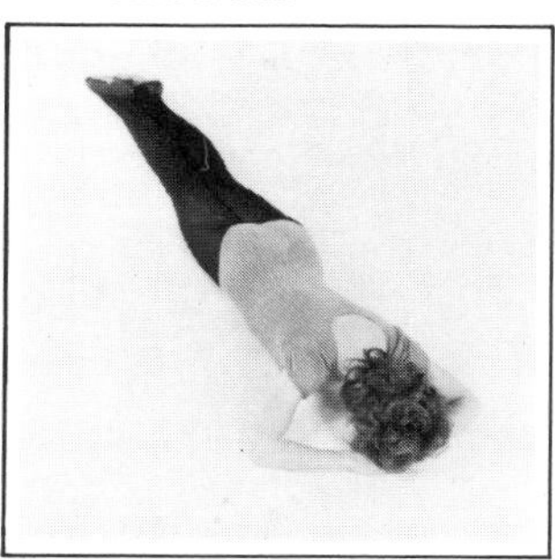

Start Lying on front, head resting on hands.
▽

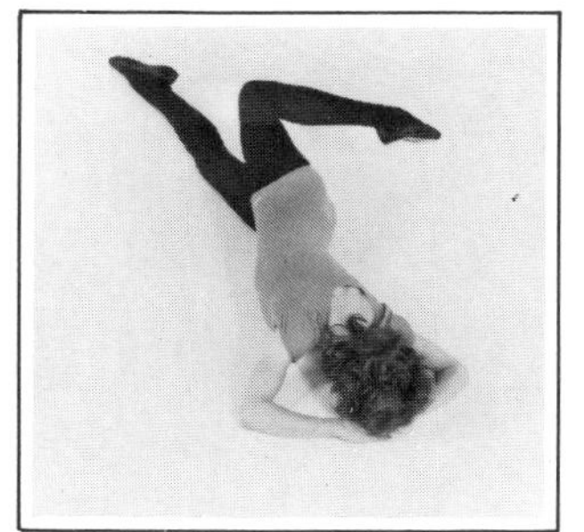

Exercise Bend one leg over the other and touch the floor.
Feel Twisted spine and firm back and buttocks.
▽

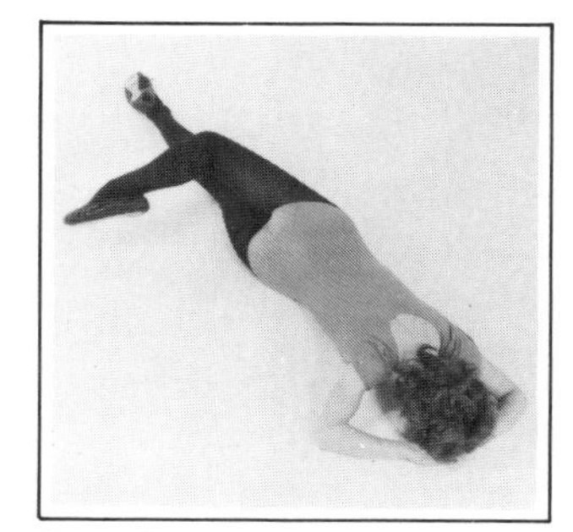

Good For Buttocks, back and spine.

Exercise Five

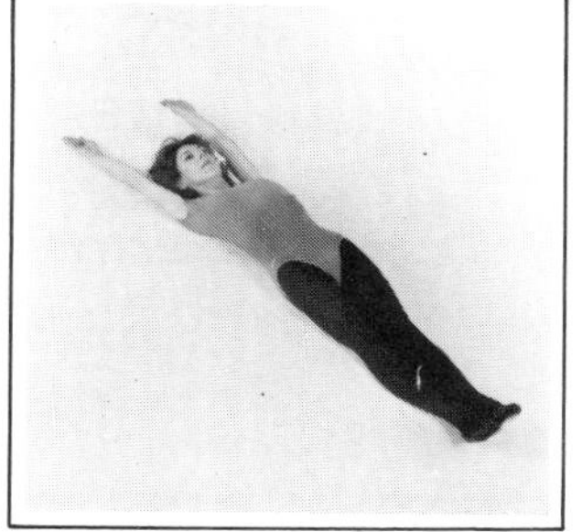

Start Lying on back, stretch arms above head.
▽

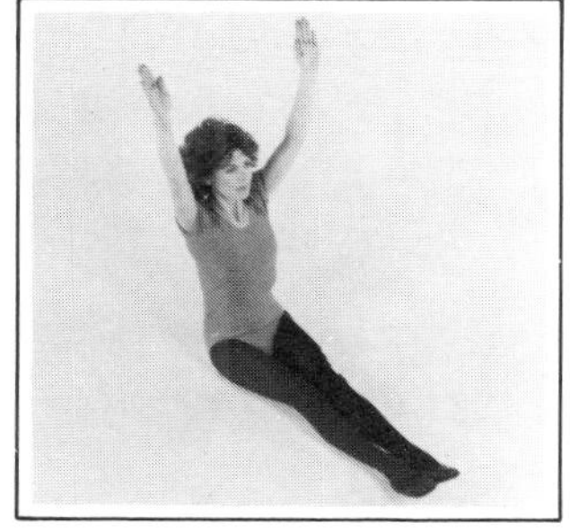

Exercise Swing arms up to sitting, relax, bend knees, straight back, reach forwards, chest towards knees.
Feel Straight strong back and stretched hips.
▽

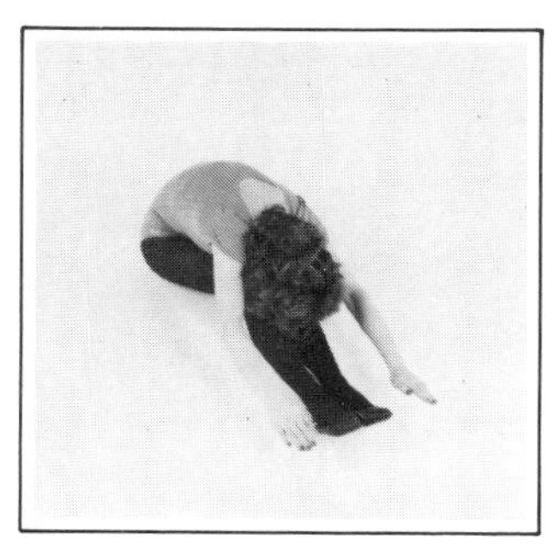

Good For Stomach and hips.

Exercise Six

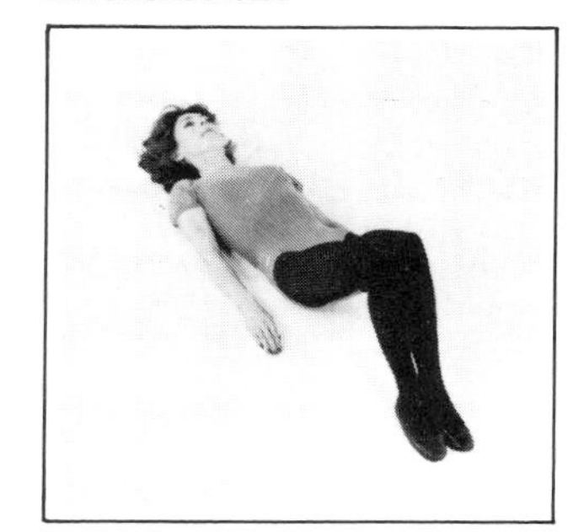

Start Crook lying.
▽

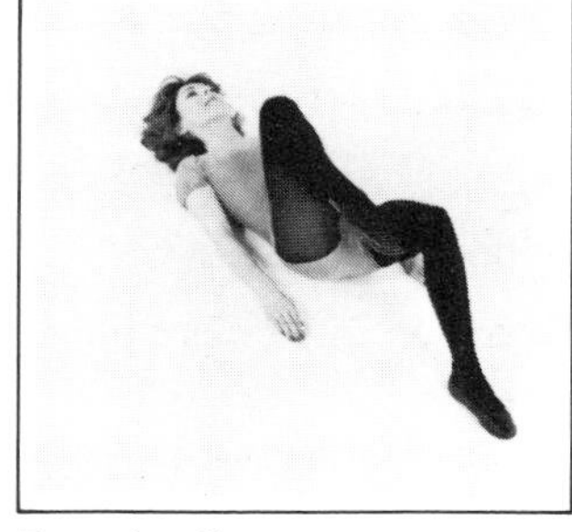

Exercise Cycle one leg at a time, keep other foot firmly on floor and still. Press back onto floor.
Feel Strong back and legs mobile.
▽

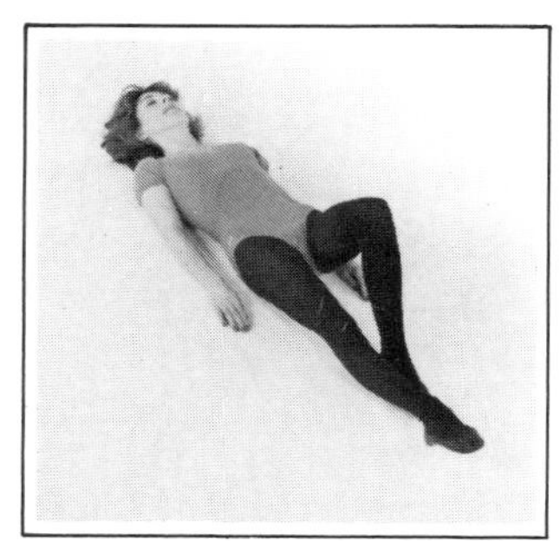

Good For Stomach and mobility of leg and hip.

THE SLIMNASTICS PROGRAMME

Week XII
Healthy Eating Programme (stock taking)

Weigh and measure again and note on the chart. If you are still over the ratio shown on the Recommended Weight Chart follow the ideas under the chapter on Obesity in Section 4.

This week do another of the menus on pp 38-9.

Go through your stock cupboard and make sure it does not contain any more unhealthy foods (such as refined starches and sugars). Look through your freezer too if you have one. In emergency you will eat what you have, make sure it will really help you and do you good.

Tension Control Technique (time off)

Continue as before. Give yourself a treat! Take a day off, do something you have been longing to have the courage or time to do for ages, just spoil yourself for a change. A touch of frivolity does wonders for the soul.

Weight this Week .... st. .... lb.

The Slimnastics Exercises

Read the Safety Guidelines on p 18.

Wear comfortable clothing. Barefeet or non-slip shoes.

Week XII Do each exercise for 1 minute.

Exercise One

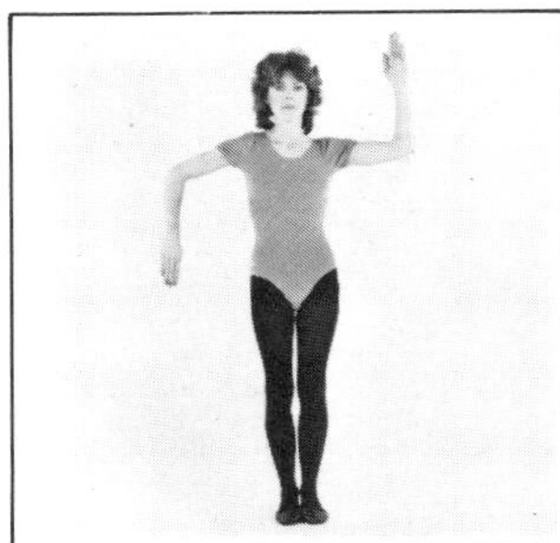

Start Standing tall, upper arms at shoulder level, head tall, one forearm up and one down.

▽

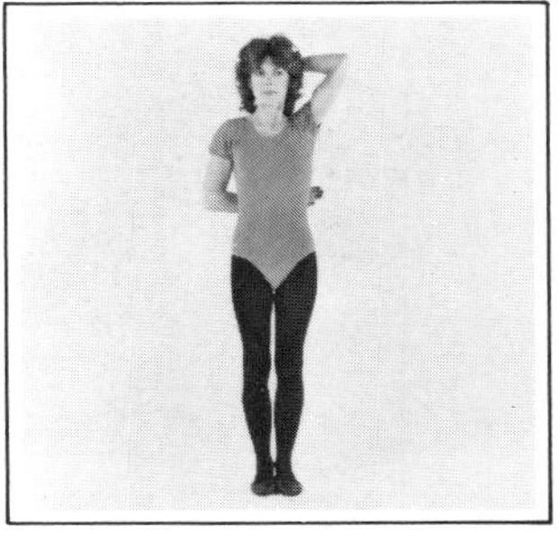

Exercise Raise one arm above head and one behind back, repeat other way.
Feel Slow movement and stretched shoulders.

▽

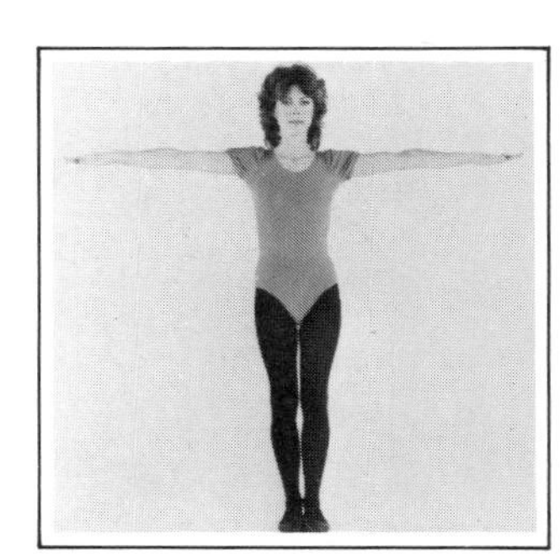

Good For Shoulder joint and blades, upper back and neck.

Exercise Two

Start Stand tall.

▽

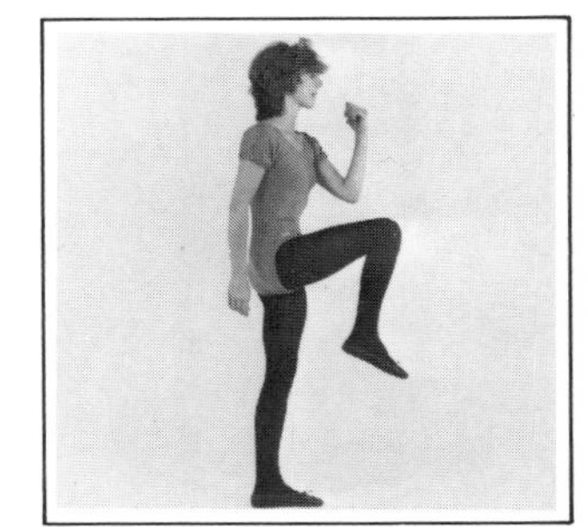

Exercise Bend alternate knee to elbow, change sides. Head up.
Feel Balanced, tall posture-twisted movement.

▽

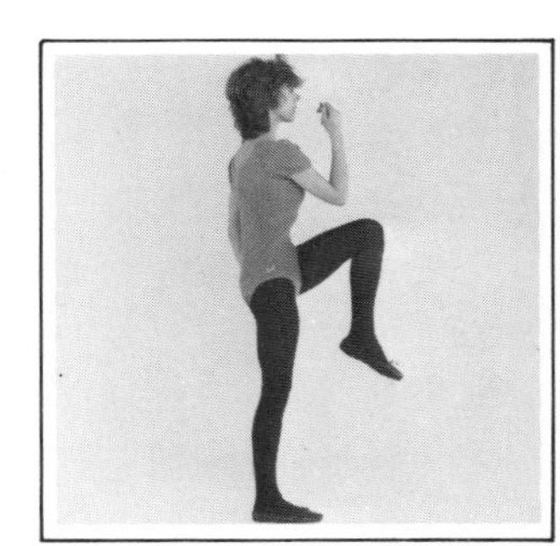

Good For Pulse, flexibility of legs, hip and waist.

WEEK 12

Exercise Three

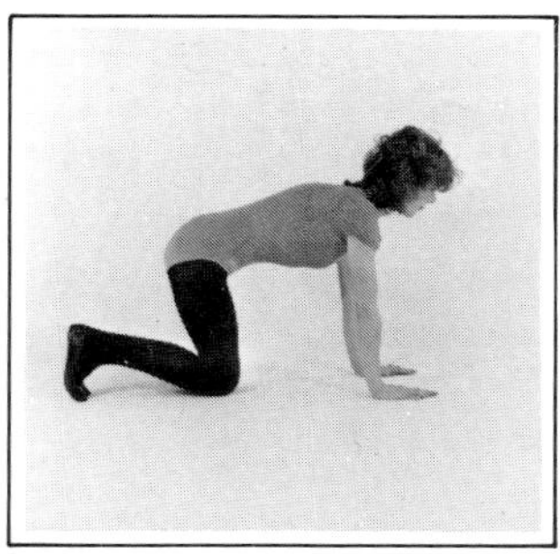

Start Prone kneeling, hands under shoulders, knees under hips.
▽

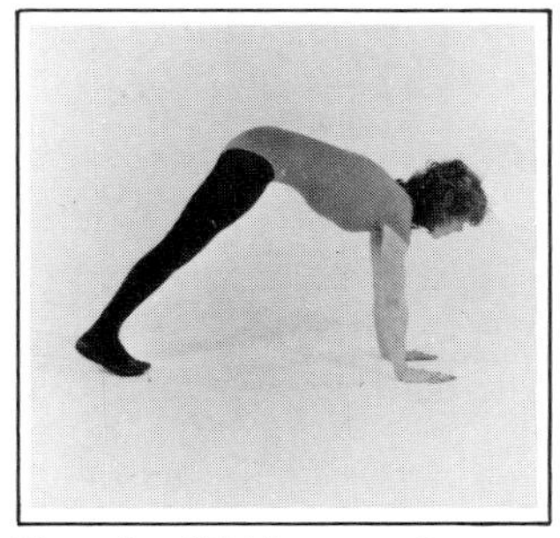

Exercise Lift hips, gently press both heels towards floor.
Feel Strong arms and double stretched legs.
▽

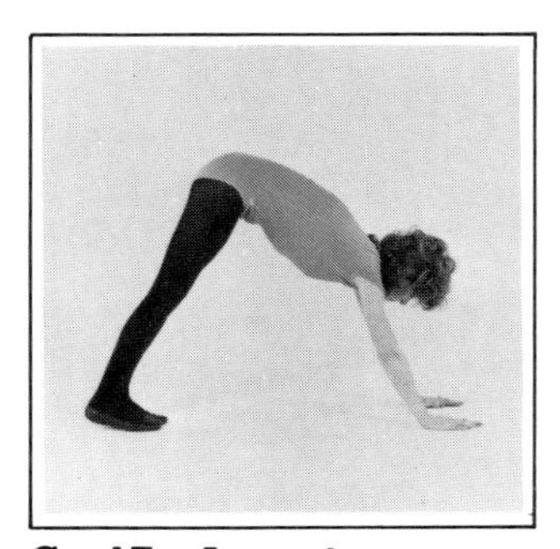

Good For Arms, chest, abdominal muscles and legs.

Exercise Four

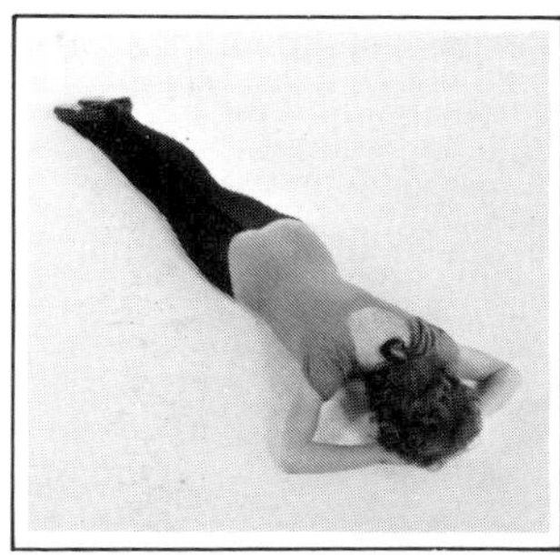

Start Lying on front, hands under head.
▽

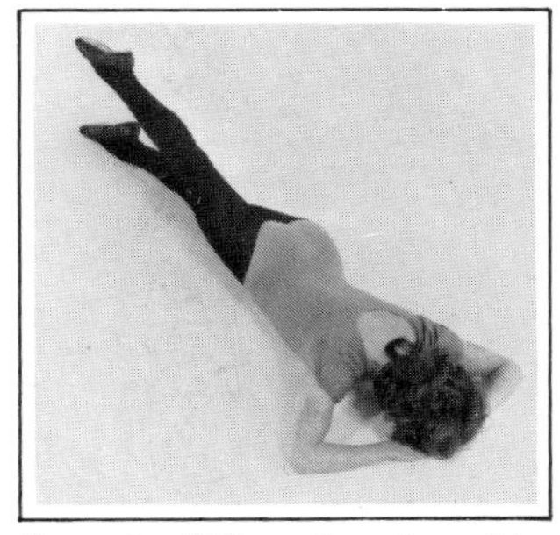

Exercise Lift one leg, from hip, keep it straight and circle clockwise then anti-clockwise, change leg.
Feel Strong and firm leg.
▽

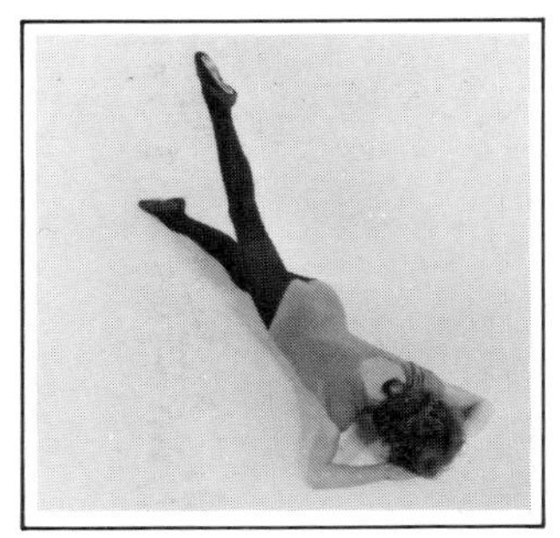

Good For Lower back, buttocks and thighs.

Exercise Five

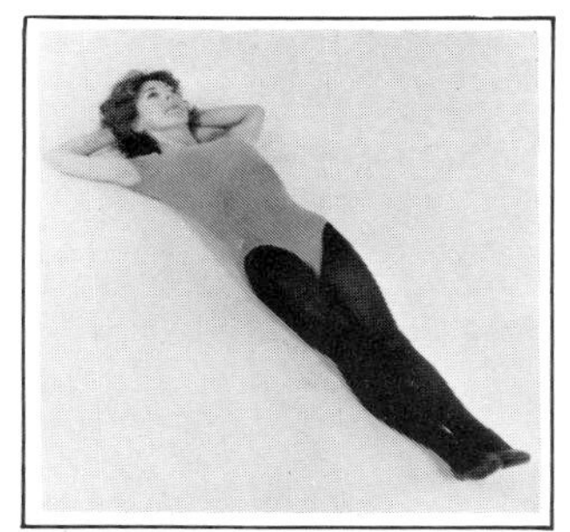

Start Lying on back, hands behind head.
▽

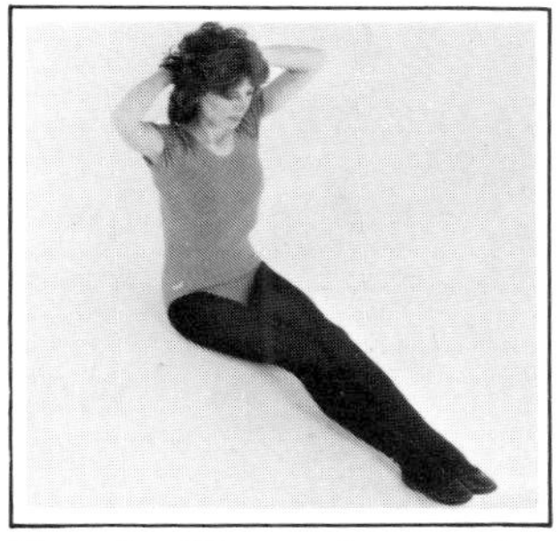

Exercise Sit up and over, relax knees, straight spine, chest towards knees.
Feel Straight, strong back and stretched hips.
▽

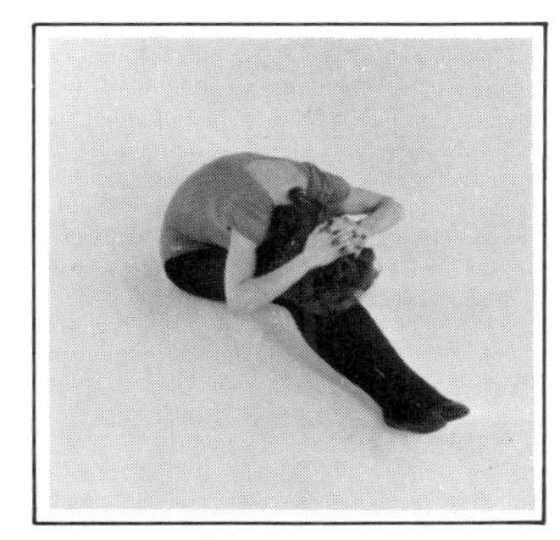

Good For Stomach and hips and arms.

Exercise Six

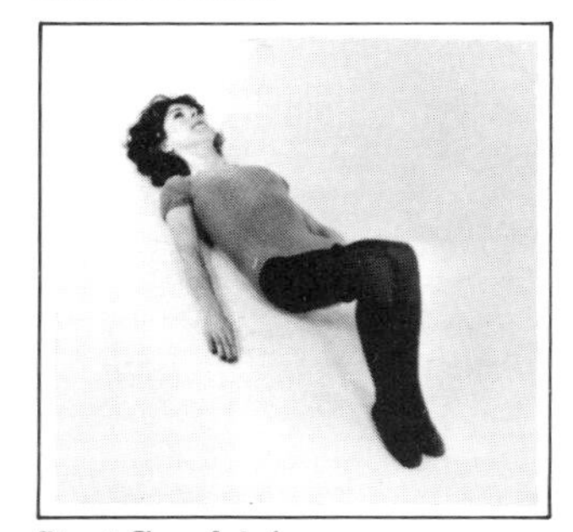

Start Crook lying.
▽

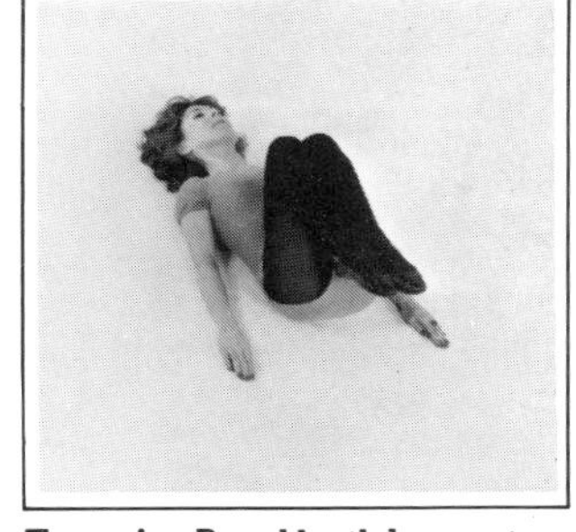

Exercise Bend both knees to chest, straighten, part, and back together. Bend. Repeat.
Feel Rhythmical movement; strong and stretched back. Press back into floor.
▽

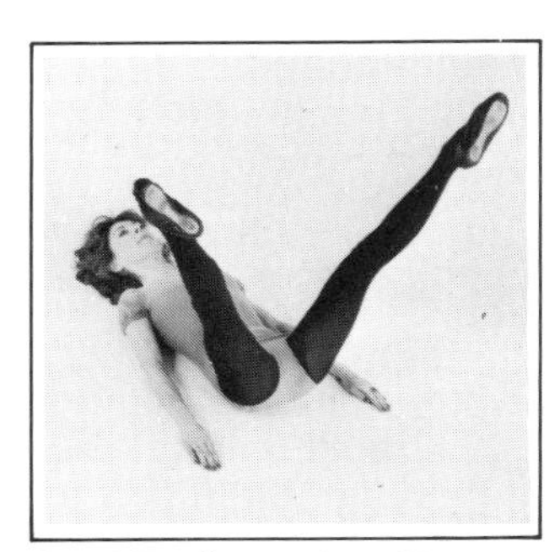

Good For Stomach and legs.

Continuation Programme

One

For the following 6 weeks ensure that the Slimnastics Programme becomes a way of life . . .

- **Eat 3 meals a day** (breakfast, a light meal and a main meal) following the Healthy Eating Programme.
- **Do Exercise Charts Weeks 1, 2, 3, 4, 5, 6, again** increasing the time for each exercise to 1½ minutes, making it a 12-minute programme.
- **Practise and use the skill of TCT** every day.
- **Take up one more form of exercise** once/twice a week.
- **Continue controlling your weight** (if necessary) limiting the alcohol (if applicable).

Two

The next 6 weeks continue as above but follow the exercise charts **Weeks 7, 8, 9, 10, 11, 12,** doing each exercise for 1½ minutes. This is a 12-minute programme. Also give up smoking (or some other form of self misuse if smoking does not apply).

Three

During the following 6 weeks, do the exercise charts in pairs i.e.

Exercise 1 of Chart A is followed by Exercise 1 of Chart B

Exercise 2 of Chart A is followed by Exercise 2 of Chart B and so on. The exercises are progressions.

The charts are paired as follows: **Weeks 1 & 2; 3 & 4; 5 & 6; 7 & 8; 9 & 10; 11 & 12.** Each exercise should be done for 1 minute. This will make a 24-minute programme. Continue the Healthy Eating and Tension Control as before plus the Take Care of Yourself Section.

Four

You can continue increasing the exercise times by doing **Weeks 1, 2, 3 & 4** together and **5, 6, 7, & 8,** followed by **9, 10, 11 & 12.** Eventually, you can complete the whole 12 doing each exercise for 1 minute. This will make a 48-minute programme.

Do not forget to continue with the Healthy Eating, the Tension Control and Living Well – all are equally important.

Your Shopping List

Your Shopping List

For your shopping list, think of including some of the following foods. Use this as a checklist and keep trying new foods or different mixtures.

Bread and Cereals

Breads
Wholemeal
Wholemeal french
Wholemeal pitta
High Bran
Wholemeal or high bran breads
Rye bread
Occasionally use other breads such as granary and fancy breads (which may not be wholemeal) to vary your diet.
Oat cakes
Pumpernickel and crispbreads
Only occasionally
Digestive or home-made biscuits

Pastas
Any type of wholewheat pasta – try the different shapes

Rice
Brown – long grain for savoury dishes, short grain for puddings or rissoles where it needs to be sticky.

Breakfast Cereals
Ideally a wholegrain cereal, with little or no added salt or sugar e.g. shredded wheat, puffed wheat, cubs or porridge oats. Otherwise use those with least added sugar and salt. Read the labels. Some bran cereals and muesli have high levels of sugar added. Some of the mueslis and crunchy cereals have added fat. Try buying your own basic ingredients to mix your own muesli.

Flour
Wholemeal plain and self-raising
Rye
Wholemeal semolina
Oatmeal or rolled oats

Vegetables – Listed fully to give you lots of ideas

Root
Jerusalem Artichokes
Beetroot
Carrots
Celeraic
Parsnips
Onions
Fennel
Garlic
Kohl Rabi
Horseradish
Leeks
Potatoes
Radishes
Turnips
Swede
Shallots
Salsify
Sweet Potato

Leafy Vegetables
Brussels sprouts
Cabbages
Spring greens
Calabrese
Red cabbage
Chicory
Broccoli
Lettuce
Chinese Leaves
Mustard and cress
Water cress
Parsley
Kale
Endive
Spinach
Swiss Chard (sea kale, beet)
Spinach beet
Bean sprouts

Other Vegetables
Globe artichokes
Asparagus
Broad beans
French beans
Runner beans
Pea beans
Celery
Cauliflower
Chicory
Marrows
Courgettes
Mushrooms
Cucumbers
Tomatoes
Peas
Endive
Pumpkin
Sweet corn
Peppers
Aubergine
Okra
Avocado Pears
Chillies
Squashes
Root ginger
Yams
Mooli

Pulses

Black eye beans
Chick peas
Flagelotes verts
Green lentils
Red lentils
Haricot beans
Mung beans
Green or yellow dried peas
Red kidney beans
Peanuts
Pinto beans
Soya beans
Aduki beans

Fruits – Also listed fully to remind you of unusual ones

Native
Apples
Crab apples
Apricots
Cherries
Greengages
Peaches
Plums
Pears
Quinces

Soft Fruits
Blackberries
Black currants
Blue berries
Bilberries
Gooseberries
Logan berries
Raspberries
Red currants
Rhubarb
Strawberries
White currants

Exotic Fruits
Bananas
Cape gooseberries
Chinese gooseberries
Cranberries
Grapes
Loquats
Lychees
Mangoes
Melons
Passion fruit
Pawpaw
Persimmons
Pineapple
Pomegranates
Kiwi fruit
Nectarines

Citrus Fruit
Clementine
Grapefruit
Kumquat
Lemon
Lime
Mandarin
Naartje
Orange
Ortanique
Satsuma
Tangerine
Ugli (tangelo)

Dried Fruits (N.B. These are high in calories)
Dates
Figs
Dried bananas
Raisins
Sultanas
Currants
Dried apricots
Dried apples
Dried pears
Dried peaches
Prunes

Nuts & Seeds (N.B. These are high in calories)

Almonds
Chestnuts
Filberts (Cobs)
Hazel nuts
Walnuts
Brazil nuts
Coconuts
Peanuts
Cashews
Mixed nuts
Sesame seeds
Sunflower seeds
Pumpkin seeds
Pine kernels
Nut butters

Fish – Again listed fully – keep experimenting

White Fish
Bass
Bream
Brill
Cod
Cod roe
Coley
Dab
Dogfish (Huss)
Flounder
Haddock
Smoked Haddock
Arbroath smokies
Hake
Halibut
Plaice
Rockfish
Skate
Sole
Lemon sole
Witch
Turbot
Whiting

Oily Fish – (N.B. These are higher in calories than white fish)
Carp
Conger eel
Common eel
Herring
Bismark herring
Bloater
Buckling
Herring roes
Kipper
Red herring
Rollmop
Salt herring
Mackerel
Smoked mackerel
Grey mullet
Red mullet
Perch
Pike
Pilchard
Salmon
Smoked salmon
Sardine
Smelt or sparling
Sprat
Rainbow trout
Brown or river trout
Sea or salmon trout
Smoked trout
Whitebait

Shellfish
Clam
Cockles
Crab
Crawfish
Lobster
Mussels
Oysters
Prawns
Scampi
Scallops
Shrimps
Whelks
Winkles

Tinned Fish (N.B. Oily fish is higher in calories)
Sardines
Mackerel
Tuna
Herring fillets
Salmon

Meat (N.B. Use the leaner cuts and smaller portions)

Beef
Veal
Lamb
Pork
Bacon
Gammon
Ham

Poultry (N.B. Duck, goose, gosling are all high in fat)
Chicken
Capon
Duck
Duckling
Goose
Gosling
Guinea fowl
Turkey

Game
Grouse
Mallard
Partridge
Pheasant
Pigeon
Quail
Snipe
Teal
Wild goose
Woodcock
Hare
Rabbit
Venison

Offal (N.B. Offal is usually cheap, high in nutrients and most are low in fat.)
Liver
Heart
Kidneys
Tongue
Brains
Sweetbreads
Tripe
Ox cheek
Black pudding

Cheeses

Cottage cheese
Curd cheese
Gouda
Edam
Brie
Camembert
Fetta
Mozzarella
Parmesan
New low-fat cheddar and cheshire cheese
(When using the higher-fat cheeses have small portions of strong flavoured varieties.)

Beverages

Mineral waters plain and sparkling
Pure orange juice*
Pure apple juice*
Pure grapefruit juice*
Pure pineapple juice*
White grape juice†
Red grape juice†
Tomato juice†
Low-calorie squash
Lemon juice
Beefy drink
Marmite
Bovril
Coffee beans
Herb Teas
Coffee
Tea
Decaffeinated coffee
Chicory
Swiss cup drink
Barley cup
Dandelion coffee
Stock cubes – low salt

*Check that no sugar is added
†Check sugar content

Snacks

Wheateats crunch
Wheateats pizza
Wheateats cheese
Wheateats natural

Oils, Dressings, Chutneys, Sauces

Olive oil
Corn oil*
Sunflower oil*
Safflower oil*
Brewers yeast
Cholesterol-free dressing
Low-calorie dressing
Mustards

*Choose a named oil for preference

Miscellaneous

Herbs
Tomato purée and pastes
Tofu (soya curd)
A few other tinned foods are useful (check sugar and salt content)
Baked beans
Tinned tomatoes
Other tinned beans for quick meals
Canned fruits in natural or apple juice

The Principal Vitamins

Common Name	Chemical Name	Good Sources	Recommended Daily Amount	What it Does For You	Deficiency Symptoms
A	Retinol	Some fatty fish, fish liver oils, margarine, animal liver, eggs, dairy produce, dark green leafy vegetables, carrots, tomatoes, apricots.	*7.50 mg Retinol equivalent	Essential for proper function of the retina. Maintains healthy skin and mucus tissue. Maybe protective against some cancer.	Poor dark adaption leading finally to blindness.
B1	Thiamine	Yeast extracts, wholemeal flour, lean meat, pulses, seeds, white bread and some cereals that are fortified.	*0.9 mg	Essential factor in carbohydrate metabolism. Important for nervous and digestive systems.	Loss of appetite, depression, loss of concentration, gastric disorders, finally beri-beri.
B2	Riboflavin	Meat and yeast extracts, liver, kidneys, meat, cheese, milk.	*1.3 mg	Important for normal growth and many enzyme systems.	Retarded or slow growth, mouth and tongue sores, poor vision, soreness of eyes.
B6	Pyridoxine	Wholegrain cereals, wheat germ, meat, fish, eggs and vegetables.	*2.0 mg	For protein metabolism.	Extra needed by those on oral contraceptives, pregnant women. Occasionally depression or neuritis.
B3	Niacin nicotinic acid, neotinamide	Bread and cereals, meat, fish, chicken, yeast extracts.	*15 mg	For healthy skin and nervous system and gastro-intestinal system.	Skin disorders, nervous and intestinal disorders. Loss of appetite, finally pellagra.
	Biotin	Liver, kidneys, yeast extracts	Unknown	Necessary for metabolism of some nutrients.	Almost unknown in man.
B5	Pantothenic acid	Yeast, liver, kidneys, egg yolk and vegetables	Suggested *5-10 mg	Release of energy from fat and carbohydrates.	Rare
B5	Folic acid	Yeast, liver, eggs, green vegetables, (easily destroyed in cooking).	*300 mg total folate	Healthy blood and rapid cell division	A type of anaemia.
B12	Cyanocobalamin	Liver, meat, yeast extracts. Only from animal origin – none from vegetable sources.	*0.3 mg	Healthy blood and nervous system.	Pernicious anaemia, degeneration of nerve cells.
C	Ascorbic acid	Fresh fruit and vegetables especially citrus fruits, black currants, tomatoes, rosehips. Easily destroyed by over-cooking.	*30 mg	Resistance to infections. For healthy connective tissues, bones, teeth and blood vessel walls.	Bleeding gums, scurvy, slow wound healing, easily bruised skin.
D	Calciferol	Sunshine on skin, margarine, oily fish, fish liver oils, eggs, butter, milk, liver.	*0.01 mg *10 mg for the elderly, children, pregnant women, lactating women	Regulates calcium and phosphorous absorption and metabolism.	Rickets and osteomalacia.
E	Tocopherol	Wheatgerm, whole grains, seeds, seed oils, milk and eggs.	Approx. 3-15 mg based on experimental evidence.	Protects body tissues. Keeps blood circulating freely.	Rare unless other diseases present.
K		Green vegetables, liver, also produced in the intestines.	Unknown.	Essential for formation of prothrombin, needed for blood clotting.	Prolonged bleeding from cuts and sores – lack of clotting agent.

*Recommended Daily Amounts of Food, Energy and Nutrients for groups of people in U.K. D.H.S.S. 1979

Vitamins are often closely linked in similar actions in the body systems. It is therefore often difficult to isolate specific effects to one vitamin. A few individuals may be more susceptible to deficiencies or have higher needs of specific vitamins. It is therefore important to consume a varied diet providing good supplies of vitamins occurring together in foods.

NOTE: Recommendations given are for groups of the population with an extra safety margin. However individual needs may vary greatly, so these can only be an approximate guide – some people will need more than these figures, some less.

The Principal Minerals

Mineral	Source	Needed for	Deficiency
Calcium	Milk, dairy foods, green vegetables, eggs, seeds, sardines,	Health of bowels, nerves and muscle. Blood clotting.	Stunted bone growth, muscle spasms.
Iron	Liver, red meats, whole grains, dried fruit, molasses and treacle. Pulses, vegetables, eggs and bread.	Needed for production of haemoglobin which transports oxygen to cells.	Lack leads to anaemia, fatigue, depression, breathlessness, skin pallor, headaches. Poor absorption; it is better from animal sources and increased if combined with Vitamin C-containing foods.
Magnesium	Cereals and vegetables.	Healthy bones, release of energy in blood cells.	Deficiency rare. Problems such as diahorrea, intestinal surgery can cause it.
Phosphorus	Almost all foods – added to some foods.	Needed with calcium for strong bones and teeth. Utilisation of energy and function of some B vitamins.	Dietary deficiency is unlikely.
Potassium	Many foods especially vegetables, meat and milk.	With sodium, balances body's water stores, so is vital to blood.	Rare in humans.
Sodium (constituent of common salt)	Almost all foods. Added to processed foods.	With potassium controls body's water balance and is essential for muscle and nerve activity.	Muscular cramps. Excess rather than deficiency is problem in Western diet, and is associated with high blood pressure.
Zinc	Nuts, legumes, seafood, meat, wholegrains. Some absorption inhibited by high phytate levels in unleavened bread and bran.	Enzyme systems concerned with nuclenic acid and protein metabolism.	Deficiency leads to: loss of appetite, impaired taste and smell, retarded growth in young, fatigue, congenital abnormalities in babies, defects in sexual organ development. Wounds will not heal normally.

The Principal Trace Elements

Trace Elements	Source	Needed for	Deficiency
Chromium	Found in wide range of food including meat and wholegrain cereals.	Proper utilisation of glucose in the body.	Rare in humans.
Cobalt		Utilised only as constituent part of Vitamin B12.	Rare in humans.
Copper	Many foods, especially green leafy vegetables, fish and liver.	Enzyme systems linked with non-metabolism in the body.	Rare in humans.
Fluoride	Drinking water in some areas, tea, fish. Added to some drinking water.	Needed for bones and teeth, increases resistance to tooth decay.	Rare in humans.
Iodine	Sea food, table salt now iodised.	Essential constituent of hormones of thyroid gland.	Enlarged thyroid gland (Goitre).
Manganese	Beans and peas, nuts, tea, wholemeal cereals.	Needed for some enzyme systems.	Rare in humans.
Molybdenum	Dependent on content of soil where food grown	Part of some enzyme systems	No deficiency shown in humans.
Nickel	Traces from utensils used in food preparation.	Traces found in body tissues but role not known.	Rare in humans.
Selenium	Cereals, nuts, seafood, meats, fruit – but depends on soil level which varies widely between areas.		Essential to function of vitamin E.
Silicon	Used as food additive. Toxic in high doses from environment e.g. quarries = silicosis.	Not clearly identified; may be required for connective tissue in man. Not yet proved to be essential.	Rare in humans.
Strontium	Same foods as calcium	Like calcium and magnesium it is stored in bone. No knowledge of role.	Deficiency not known.
Sulphur	In all proteins.	Present in protein, but role not fully understood. Two known B vitamins, thiamin and biotin, contain sulphur.	Deficiency not known.
Tin	Most comes from the tin or tin foil used in processed foods.	Trace element, used for formation of DNA and RNA, controllers of growth and hereditary characteristics.	Deficiency not known in man.
Vanadium	Wholegrain, nuts, root vegetables.		Deficiency not known, recently reported that deficiency leads to impaired growth in rats, and dental caries. May be a link with blood cholesterol levels.

Do you get enough minerals and vitamins from food?

1. Do you avoid processed foods? And choose natural unrefined ones?
2. Are you careful that the vegetables and fruit that you eat are not stored for a long time, pre-soaked, over-cooked or kept hot? And that vegetables do not have salt added?
3. Do you eat a wide range of different foods? Regularly?
4. Do you eat some fresh vegetables and fresh fruit every day?
5. Are you female? And under the age of the menopause and over the age of puberty?
6. Where do you live?

If you answered 'yes' to questions 1-4, you are giving yourself the best chance of getting a good supply of minerals from food.

However, if you are a woman in her child-bearing years, you still need to watch out for one particular mineral: iron. Iron, is the mineral that many women have a poor supply of – or absorb poorly.

Women need more than men, especially if they have many children or heavy periods.

Question 6 is the one that really marks a difference between minerals and vitamins. For while vitamins are evenly produced by plants and in animals, minerals vary in different soils. If a mineral is low in certain soil, it will also be low in the produce grown there; the plants cannot make it.

N.B. Those who are most at risk of deficiency are those who

- Eat a limited or 'fad' diet
- Have a high proportion of processed foods in their diet
- Suffer from diseases affecting their digestion or absorption of foods

Additives

Packet soups, stock cubes and meat spreads contain many sodium additives. Most confectionery contains a whole range of dyes, including the doubtful tartrazine. Any food which is highly coloured (and therefore appeals more to children) will probably be artificially dyed. Tartrazine also figures in fizzy drinks and sugary squashes. It's worth remembering too, that processed meat may contain added fat and stabiliser to bulk it out, and that 'succulent' pre-packed ham probably looks so juicy because it has been injected with water-holding phosphates.

Taken from *Look at the Label*, the following are a selection of some of the most common serial numbers which can be used on food labels as alternatives to the specific names of additives.

E 101	Riboflavin or Lactoflavin
E 102	Tartrazine
E 141	Copper complexes of chlorophyll and chlorophyllins
E 142	Green S or Acid Brilliant Green BS or Lissamine Green
E 150	Caramel
E 201	Sodium sorbate
E 202	Potassium sorbate
E 203	Calcium Sorbate
E 210	Benzoic acid
E 211	Sodium benzoate
E 213	Potassium benzoate
E 213	Calcium benzoate
E 221	Sodium sulphite
E 222	Sodium hydrogen sulphite
E 223	Sodium metabisulphite
E 232	Sodium biphenyl-2-yl oxide
E 236	Formic acid
E 237	Sodium formate
E 239	Hexamine
E 249	Potassium nitrate
E 250	Sodium nitrate
E 251	Sodium nitrate
E 252	Potassium nitrate
E 260	Acetic acid
E 262	Sodium hydrogen diacetate
E 270	Lactic acid
E 280	Propionic acid
E 281	Dodium propionate
E 290	Carbon dioxide
E 300	L-Ascorbic acid
E 301	Sodium-L-ascorbate
E 320	Butylated hydroxyanisole
E 321	Butylated hydroxytoluene
E 322	Lecithins
E 325	Sodium lactate
E 326	Potassium lactate
E 330	Citric acid
E 331	Sodium dihydrogen citrate
E 331	diSodium citrate
E 331	triSodium citrate
E 332	Potassium dihydrogen citrate
E 332	Potassium citrate
E 333	Calcium citrate
E 333	diCalcium citrate
E 333	triCalcium citrate
E 334	Tartaric acid
E 335	Sodium tartrate
E 336	Potassium tartrate
E 336	Potassium hydrogen tartrate
E 337	Potassium sodium tartrate
E 339(a)	Sodium dihydrogen orthophosphate
E 339(b)	diSodium hydrogen orthophosphate
E 339(c)	triSodium orthophosphate
E 401	Sodium alginate*
E 402	Potassium alginate*
E 403	Ammonium alginate*
E 404	Calcium alginate
E 414	Acacia or Gum Arabic
E 420(i)	Sorbitol
E 420(ii)	Sorbitol syrup
E 421	Mannitol
E 422	Gylcerol
E 440(a)	Pectin
E 440(b)	Pectin, amidated
E 450(a)	diSodium dihydrogen diphosphate
E 450(a)	tetraSodium diphosphate
E 450(a)	tetra Potassium diphosphate
E 450(a)	triSodium diphosphate
E 450(b)	pentaSodium triphosphate
E 450(b)	pentaPotassium triphosphate
E 450(c)	Sodium polyphosphates
E 450(c)	Potassium polyphosphates
E 461	Methylcellulose
E 463	Hydroxypropyl-cellulose
E 464	Hydroxypropyl-methylcellulose
E 465	Ethylmethylcellulose
E 466	Carboxymethyl-cellulose sodium salt
E 470	Sodium, potassium and calcium salts of fatty acids
E 471	Mono-and di-glycerides of fatty acids
E 481	Sodium stearoyl-2-lactylate

Herbs and Their Culinary Uses

HERB		CULINARY USE
Angelica	Stems	Crystallised for decorating cakes and desserts.
	Leaves	Chopped, for salads or fresh fruit.
Anise	Seeds	Tiny amounts flavour rye bread, cheese biscuits.
Apple Mint	Leaves	Refreshing with fruit sorbets (sherbets).
Basil	Leaves	Flavour soups, egg dishes, vegetables, salads and dressings, fish, poultry, pork and veal. Pounded with garlic as a sauce.
Bay	Leaves	Valuable in stews, sauces, soups, pâtés, and stuffings and in fish dishes.
Bergamot	Leaves and flowers	Chopped in salads and pork dishes.
Borage	Flowers	To decorate wine cups.
	Leaves	Chopped in salads, salad dressings, egg dishes; use with cucumber.
Caraway	Seeds	Tiny amounts flavour rye bread, cheese biscuits (crackers) and some potato dishes.
Chervil	Leaves	Delicate flavour enhances chicken, fish, veal, salads, egg dishes, tomatoes. Basis of soup.
Chives	Leaves	Lose flavour when cooked. Garnish for soups, eggs, fish, chicken and veal; use with salads and vegetables.
Comfrey	Leaves	Chopped for salads; cooked like spinach; young leaves can be dipped in batter and eaten as fritters.
Coriander	Seeds	Crushed; especially with curries and pickles. Flavouring for soups, pâtés, fish, poultry, game, lamb, pork, vegetables and sauces.
	Leaves	Add spicy hot taste when chopped and added to curries after cooking.
Cumin	Seeds	Combines with coriander to flavour vegetable dishes and curries.
Dill	Leaves	Excellent with fish, chicken, rabbit, veal and salads. Goes well with mustard.
	Seeds & stems	Used for pickling
Marshmallow	Leaves & tops	Chopped, in salads.

HERB		CULINARY USE
Nasturtium	Leaves	Add peppery taste to salads and sandwiches.
	Flowers	Garnish for salad.
	Seeds	Pickled – use like capers.
Parsley	Leaves & Stalks	Flavour all savoury dishes, hot or cold; as a garnish; in sauces; basis of salad, deep fried as a garnish.
Peppermint	Leaves	Flavour fruit salads, summer drinks and sorbets. Use for peppermint syrup.
Purslane	Leaves	Chopped in salads and dressings with egg dishes and vegetables.
	Young shoots	Lightly boiled and served as a vegetable.
Rose	Hips	Cooked with sugar for syrups, sauces, jellies.
Rosemary	Leaves	With all meat, particularly roast lamb, in stuffings and marinades.
Sage	Leaves	Flavour pâtés and stuffings, egg dishes, poultry and game, pork, veal and vegetables (especially onions), sauces and dressings.
Salad Burnet	Leaves	Delicate flavour best with creamy sauces, salads, white meats, egg dishes, tomato and cucumber.
Spearmint	Leaves	Chopped in vegetable dishes, in mint sauce as a sauce with garlic and yoghurt, with salads.
Summer Savory	Leaves	Chopped in stuffings and sausages, with game.
Sweet Cicely	Leaves	Chopped with cooked fruit. Add to water when cooking cabbage.
Tarragon	Leaves	Best with chicken, fish and eggs. Chopped in sauces and as a herb butter.
Thyme	Leaves	All savoury dishes, especially veal, chicken, game and in tomato sauce.
Watercress	Leaves & stems	Basis for hot or cold soups, in salads, garnish for steaks.
Woodruff	Leaves & stems	Partially dried and added to apple juice, wine and cider cups.
Elder	Flowers	Flavour sorbets, jams, jellies, and vinegars.
	Berries	Make wine, jams and jellies.
Fennel	Leaves	Best with fish, also in soups and stuffings or with pork.
	Seeds	Flavour stuffings for fish.

HERB		CULINARY USE
Garlic	Bulbs (Cloves)	Flavour all savoury dishes hot or cold.
Hops	Shoots	Lightly boiled and served as a vegetable.
Horseradish	Root	Grated into sauce for hot or cold roast beef, braised beef or smoked fish.
Hyssop	Leaves	Use sparingly when roasting duck, goose or pork, and in rich pâtés.
Juniper	Berries	Crushed into marinades; flavour stuffings for game and pâtés.
Lemon Balm	Leaves	Chopped in salad dressings, soups, sauces and chicken dishes.
Lemon Thyme	Leaves	Fish dishes.
Lemon Verbena	Leaves	Very strong lemon flavouring for fresh fruit salads and summer drinks.
Lovage	Leaves	Celery-like flavour excellent in all savoury dishes, hot or cold.
	Seeds	Flavour stuffings, pâtés and stews.
Marigold	Flower	Add flavour and colour to soups, beef stews.
	Petals	Salads and cheese dishes.
Marjoram	Leaves	Flavour game, beef and chicken dishes, sausages and tomatoes.

Spices and Their Culinary Uses

SPICE	CULINARY USE
Allspice	Meatballs, cranberry dishes, pickles, relishes, asparagus; vegetable, beef, pea and minestrone soups; fruit salads, cottage cheese, beets, spinach, turnips, carrots, beef, ham, lamb, fish, fruit compote and apples.
Caraway Seed	Soft cheese spreads, most soups, cole slaw and salads, sauerkraut, beets, cabbage, turnips, asparagus, potatoes, tomatoes, cottage cheese, omelettes, pork, liver, kidneys, sauerbraten, goulash, roast goose and tuna casseroles.
Cardamom Seed	Pea soup, fruit salads, oranges and grapefruits, beef, sausages, pork, bread and fruit cups.
Cayenne or Red Pepper & Cayenne	Devilled recipes, avocado dips, chowders, oyster stew, tuna, chicken, shrimp, meat, macaroni salads, eggs, cottage cheese, welsh rarebit, cheese souffles, pork, veal, beef, pasta dishes, oysters, shell fish and chicken.
Celery Salt, flakes, seeds	Sauerkraut, tomato juice, ham spread, pickles, most soups, fish chowders, bouillion, salad dressings, cole slaw, potato salads, egg and tuna salads, turnips, cauliflower, cabbage, potatoes, stewed tomatoes, eggs, rarebit, meat loaf, meat stews, pot roasts, chicken, stuffings and fish.
Chilli Powder & Pepper	Avocado dips, pepperpot, corn soup, chowders, tomato soup, chilli, fresh dressings, kidney bean salads, corn Mexicall, carrots, eggplant, green peas, rice, tomatoes, eggs, omelettes, casseroles, cheese, rarebits, soufflés, Mexican dishes, meat loaf, beef, hamburgers, stews, seafoods and chicken.
Cinnamon	Gherkins, cinnamon toast, heated spiced beverages, fruit salad, sweet potatoes, pumpkin, spinach, pork, ham, lamb, chicken and some fish dishes, breads, baked apples and stewed fruits.
Cloves	Fruit punch, gherkins, hot spiced wines, lean beef, tomato and pea soups, topping for fruit salad, beets, baked beans, sweet potatoes, ham or roast pork, stews, tongue, sausages, baked fish, chicken dishes and pickled or stewed fruits.
Curry Powder	Tomato juice, pickles, dips, chowders, tomato or mushroom soups, creamed vegetables, rice, tomatoes, eggs, cottage cheese, veal, lamb and beef dishes.
Ginger	Grilled grapefruit, pickles; bean, onion and potato soup; topping for fruit salad, beets, carrots, baked beans, egg and cheese dishes, beef, lamb, veal, chicken, fish, stewed or preserved fruits.
Mace	Chicken soup, spinach, mashed potatoes, cheese dishes, lamb, veal, meat loaf, chicken, fish and fruit salad.
Mixed Spice	Pickling preserves, stewed apples and melon.
Mustard Seed	Pickles, ham spread, bean and onion soups, salad garnishes and salads, broccoli, asparagus, baked beans, Brussels sprouts, cabbage, beets, potatoes, cheese sauces, eggs, casseroles, pickled meat, ham, kidneys, oysters, shrimps and fish.
Nutmeg	Chopped oysters; chicken, mushroom and vegetable beef soups; salad dressings, steamed and glazed carrots, cabbage, spinach, cauliflower, sweet potatoes, cheese sauces, fondue, meat loaf, most chicken dishes, stewed fruit and egg nog.
Pickling Spice	Pickled relishes, beef broth soup, baked cabbage, boiled beets, sauerkraut, pickling, stews, pork, veal, lamb, beef, shrimps, fish and game.
Poppy Seed	Dips, onion soup, most salad dressings, peas, potatoes, sweet potatoes, carrots, cottage cheese, scrambled eggs, omelettes and noodle dishes.
Sesame Seeds	Soft cheeses, most soups, dressings, spinach, tomatoes, noodle and vegetable dishes, casseroles, asparagus, potato and rice dishes, fish and chicken dishes.

Daily Diet Record

Daily Food & Drink for One Week							
DAY	BREAKFAST	11 am	LUNCH	TEA	SUPPER/DINNER	DRINKS/SNACKS	PARTIES/ILLNESS/EXCUSES!

Slimnastics Weight Graph

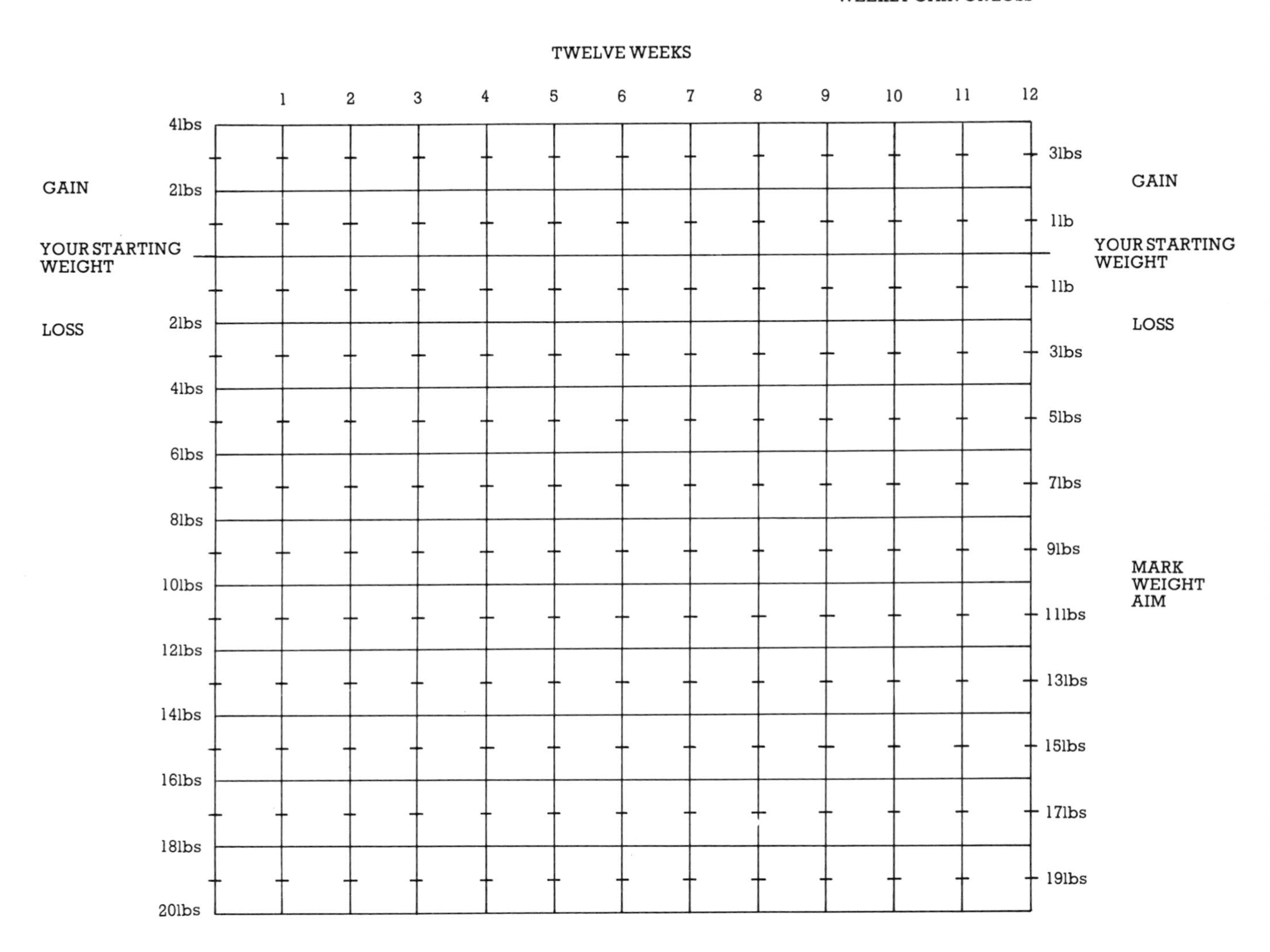

Bibliography

Dental Caries – Aetiology, Pathology and Prevention; Silverstone, Johnson, Handrie, Williams; Macmillan Press Ltd, 1981.
Stress and Relaxation; Jane Madders; Martin Dunitz.
Living with Stress; *Which Report*: a Consumer Publication
Simple Relaxation; Laura Mitchell; John Murray.
The Principles of Exercise Therapy (3rd Edition); M. Dena Gardiner; Bell.
Anatomy of the Human Body; Lochhart, Hamilton and Fyfe; Faber and Faber.
Function of the Human Body (3rd Edition); A.G. Guyton; Saunders.
Anatomy and Ballet; Celia Spayer; Black.
Salt in the Diet; The British Nutrition Foundation Briefing Paper; June 1981.
British Food Journal, 'Diet and Blood'; May/June 1983.
Prevention and Health 'Drinking Well'; Dept. of Health and Social Security Health Education Council; H.M.S.O.
Smoking among Secondary School Children; Offices of Population Censuses and Surveys; Health Education Council, 1983.
Obesity; Royal College of Physicians Report, R.C.P. 1983.
Putting Good Nutrition into Practice; Donald W. Sarll, MDS, BDS; Prize-winning paper in the 1982 Van den Berghs & Jurgens Nutrition Award.
Prescription for a Better British Diet; R. Passmore, Dorothy F. Hollingsworth, Jean Robertson; British Medical Journal, 1979.
Look at the Label; Booklet by the Ministry of Agriculture, Fisheries and Food; H.M.S.O.
What are Children Eating these Days?; National Dairy Council, 1982.
Report on Medical Aspects of Dietary Fibre 1980; Royal College of Physicians; Pitman.
Which Report, 'Prevention of CHD'; 1982.
Eating for Health; DHSS 1979.
Implementation of Dietary Guidelines, Obstacles and Opportunities; British Nutrition Foundation, 1982.
Changing Food Habits in the U.K.; Chris Wardle; Earth Resources Research Publication, 1977.
Taking the Rough with the Smooth; Andrew Stanway; Pan Books.
Don't Forget Fibre in Your Diet; Denis Burkett; Martin Dunitz.
The Diabetics Diet Book; John Mann and the Oxford Diabetic Group; Martin Dunitz.
The Right Way to Eat; Mirriam Polurin.

For further information:
Health Education Council
British Nutrition Foundation
British Medical Council
The Sports Council of Great Britain and Central Council for Physical Recreation
The Slimnastics Organisation

Diana Lamplugh and Pamela Nottidge founded Slimnastics in 1964 since which time it has grown into an organisation with 300 fully trained leaders and a membership of over 25,000. Demand exceeds the number of places and both the numbers of leaders and members are still expanding.
Diana Lamplugh has studied teaching methods, relaxation techniques and psychology, and currently teaches Slimnastics at two London colleges, trains Slimnastics tutors, assesses all Slimnastics leaders and teaches swimming. Pamela Nottidge has a Diploma in the Theory and Practice of Physical Education and currently teaches students at St Thomas' Hospital, the Nightingale School of Nurses and the Lambeth Health Education Authority; she also lectures and runs Slimnastics classes for doctors, dentists and teachers.

Other books by the same authors
Slimnastics (Angus & Robertson, 1970)
(Penguin, 1971)
Stress and Overstress (Angus & Robertson, 1970)
The New Penguin Slimnastics (Penguin, 1980)